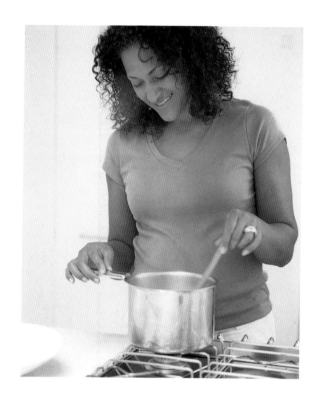

feel-good foods
for pregnancy

D1300645

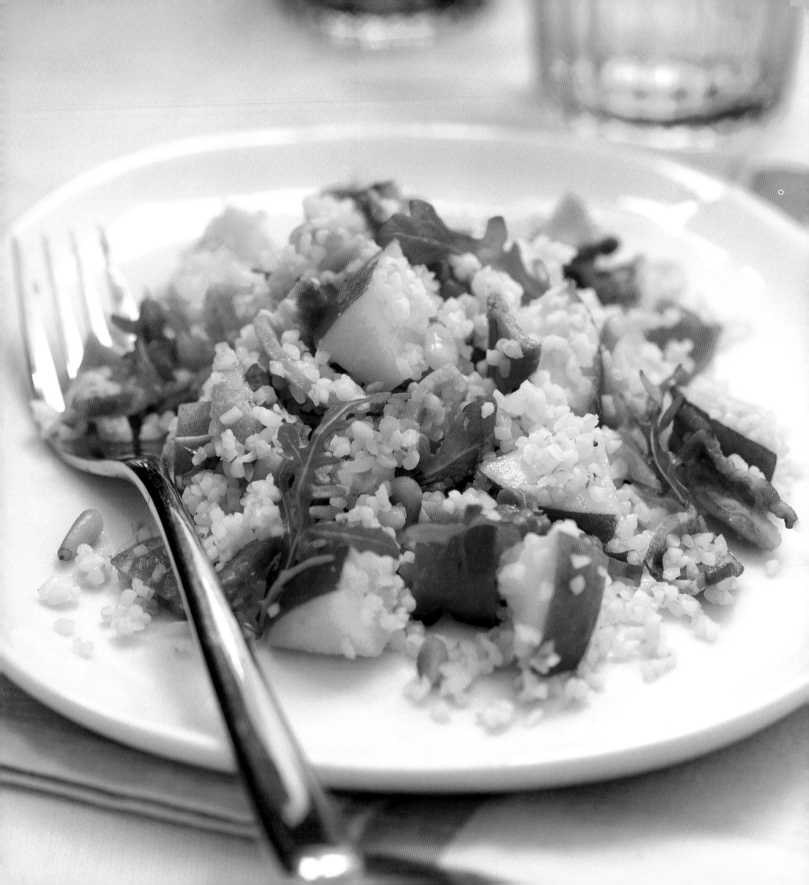

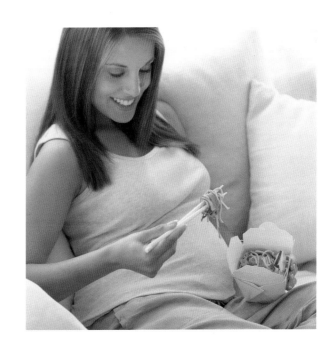

feel-good foods
for pregnancy

lyndel costain and nicola graimes

with photography by william reavell
and winfried heinze

RYLAND
PETERS
& SMALL

LONDON NEW YORK

Notes All spoon measurements are level, unless otherwise specified. Ovens should be preheated to the specified temperature. Recipes in this book were tested using a regular oven. If using a convection oven, follow the manufacturer's instructions for adjusting temperatures. All eggs are medium, unless otherwise specified.

Neither the authors nor the publisher can be held responsible for any claim arising out of the use or misuse of the information in this book. Always consult your healthcare professional or doctor if you have any concerns about your health or nutrition.

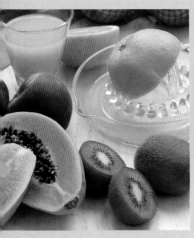

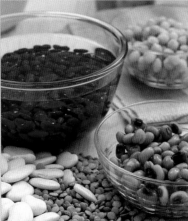

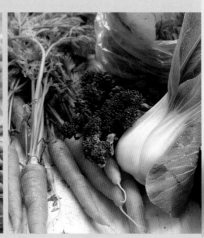

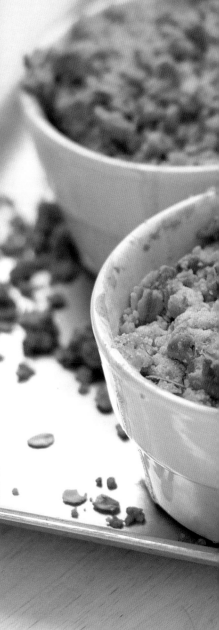

Senior Designer Toni Kay
Senior Editor Catherine Osborne
Production Gemma John
Location Research Jess Walton
Art Director Leslie Harrington
Publishing Director Alison Starling

US Consultant Theresa C Kinsella
Food Stylists Annie Rigg and Libby Rea Brownlee
Stylist Liz Belton
Make-up Artist Marie Coulter
Indexer Ann Barrett

First published in the United States
in 2008 by Ryland Peters & Small, Inc.
519 Broadway, 5th Floor
New York, NY 10012
www.rylandpeters.com

10 9 8 7 6 5 4 3 2 1

Text © Lyndel Costain and Nicola Graimes 2008
Design and photographs
© Ryland Peters & Small 2008

Printed in China

ISBN 978 1 84597 586 9

Library of Congress Cataloging-in-Publication Data

Costain, Lyndel.
  Feel-good foods for pregnancy / Lyndel Costain and Nicola Graimes with photography by William Reavell and Winfried Heinze.
      p. cm.
  Includes index.
  ISBN 978-1-84597-586-9
  1. Pregnancy--Nutritional aspects. 2. Mothers--Nutrition. 3. Cookery. I. Graimes, Nicola. II. Title.
  RG559.C67 2008
  641.5'6319--dc22
                                    2007043316

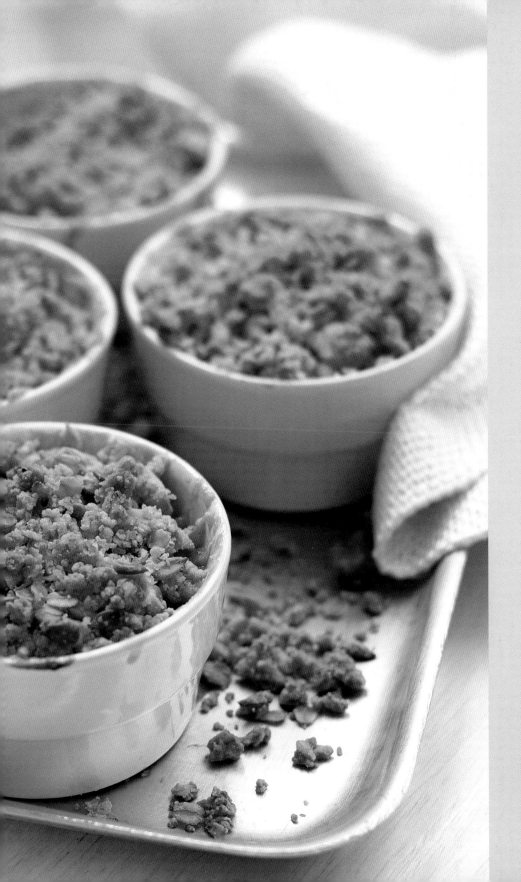

contents

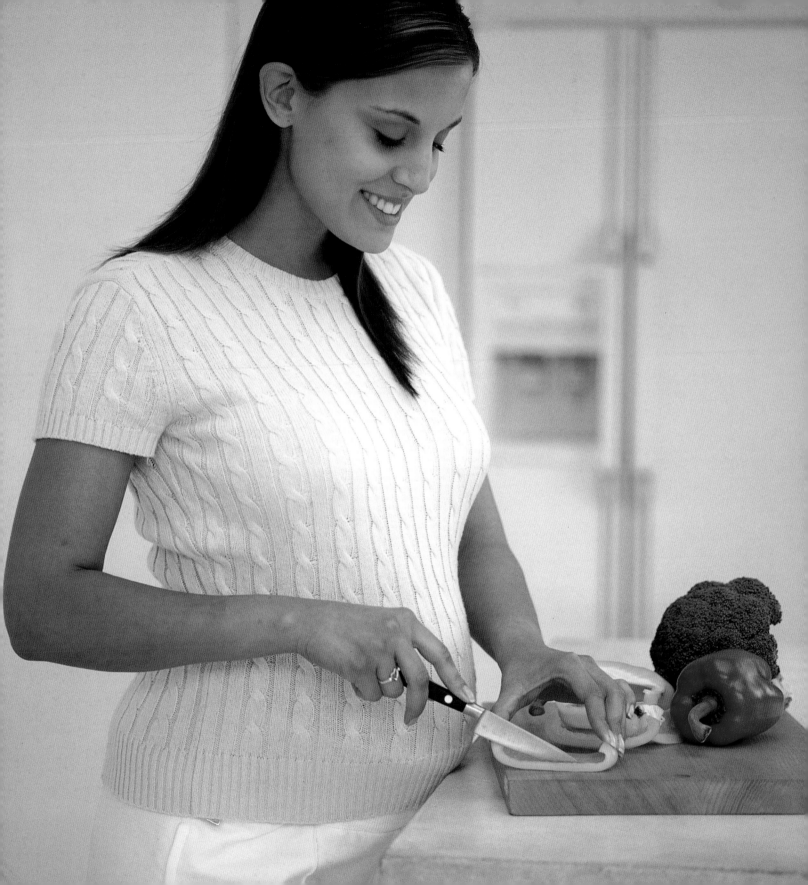

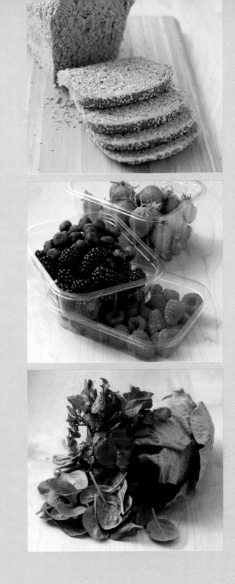

YOUR HEALTHY PREGNANCY

Planning a baby?

If you are planning to have a baby, it is the time to examine your, and your partner's, diet and lifestyle. You may decide to make a number of changes before you start trying to conceive. There is good evidence that not smoking and being well nourished at the time of conception is important for the health and development of your baby, including their future adult health. Not only does it increase the chance of the successful fertilization of a healthy egg and sperm, but provides the best environment to support the immediate, and very rapid, growth of your baby. By the third week after conception, the embryo has already started to develop a heart, brain, and spinal cord, and by the eighth week, the structural foundations of the body have been laid down. This rapid building of new cells requires an adequate supply of nutrients including protein, fats, vitamins, and minerals, which are the essential building blocks of a new life.

PREPARING FOR A BABY

○ **Enjoy a healthy balanced diet** Consuming a variety of foods before you conceive will provide you with the critical nutrients needed to nourish your body during pregnancy, especially during the early stages when morning sickness may prevent you from eating well. It also helps you stay fit and healthy.

○ **Women should not drink alcohol while they are pregnant or planning to become pregnant** Alcohol passes from the blood stream and through the placenta to your unborn baby. Alcohol consumption increases the risk of fetal alcohol syndrome, impaired fetal growth, and may reduce fertility.

○ **If you smoke, work to stop** You no doubt know that smoking is bad for your health, and it harms your baby. It can also make it harder to conceive and increases the risk of miscarriage. Many people—both women and their partners—find this is the ideal time to finally quit. Enlist support from family, friends, health professionals, or local support groups. Also avoid secondhand smoke whenever possible.

○ **Aim to be a healthy weight** Starting pregnancy at a healthy body weight (*see* Body Mass Index chart on page 11) makes conception more likely and improves pregnancy outcomes. Being underweight can make it more difficult to conceive, as low weight upsets the production of hormones essential for normal menstruation and ovulation. It also increases the risk of your baby being born early or having a low birth weight (see page 9). Being overweight can also affect ovulation and therefore conception.

Women who are overweight are more likely to develop complications such as high blood pressure and diabetes during pregnancy. There's also an increased chance of delivering early, as well as the possibility of requiring a Caesarean section. If you feel you would benefit from losing some weight, combine a healthy calorie-controlled diet with regular exercise. To ensure you are well nourished when you do become pregnant, resist any temptation to crash diet. Focus on losing just one to two pounds a week. Losing just five to ten percent of your weight can make a real difference. Talk to your doctor if you need help.

○ **Pay attention to your iron intake** Iron is needed to help make cells, including red blood cells. A lack of iron can deplete iron stores in the body and lead to energy-sapping iron deficiency and anemia. Starting off with good iron stores is vital for a healthy pregnancy (*see* page 14). Some women are more at risk of being iron deficient and may require iron supplements. Talk to your doctor if you have very heavy monthly blood losses, are a teenager, or had a baby less than a year ago.

○ **Check any medications, ointments, herbal remedies, or nutritional supplements** Talk to your doctor, midwife, pharmacist, or herbal practitioner to see whether or not they are safe to start using or continue to use. Take a 400-microgram (mcg) supplement of folic acid daily. Folic acid is a B vitamin that helps to prevent babies being born with neural-tube defects such as spina bifida. It is recommended that all women planning pregnancy take this supplement, and continue until their 12th week of pregnancy. If you are taking a prenatal supplement (*see* page 21), it should contain 400 mcg folic acid. You should also eat plenty of foods containing folic acid (*see* pages 15–16).

○ **Start to follow pregnancy food hygiene and food safety advice** Avoid liver and foods that carry a risk of causing food poisoning from listeria, salmonella, and toxoplasmosis such as blue, unpasteurized and mold-ripened soft cheeses, pâté, raw or undercooked meat, fish, and eggs. Take care to store and prepare food safely (*see* page 28).

○ **See your doctor about any existing health problems** If you have any health problems, talk to your doctor so you can understand how pregnancy may affect them. You can then ensure you plan ahead for the best medical care.

○ **Enjoy daily walks or other regular physical activity** Regular physical activity is an important part of a healthy lifestyle. It also helps boost your energy levels and immune system and manage your weight and stress levels. You don't need to be an athlete. Fitting in at least 30 minutes of moderately intense activity, such as brisk walking, gardening, cycling, swimming, or dancing, at least five times a week, is enough to benefit your health.

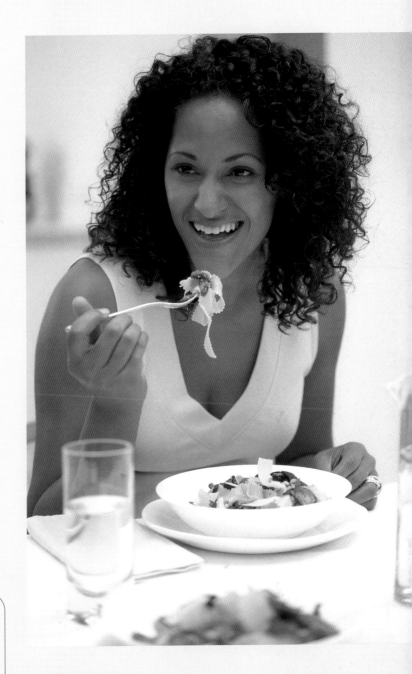

Birth weight

A baby born with a good birth weight has a far lower chance of getting sick as a baby, or having physical, learning, or behavioral problems. It may also benefit their long-term health, for example reduce their risk of type 2 diabetes or early heart disease. Many factors can influence birth weight. Research shows that not smoking, good nutrition, and not being underweight before and during pregnancy are key factors that help to ensure a healthy birth weight.

Note: If you are already pregnant and have just read the advice on this page, don't worry. It is not too late for you and your baby to benefit from a healthy diet and lifestyle.

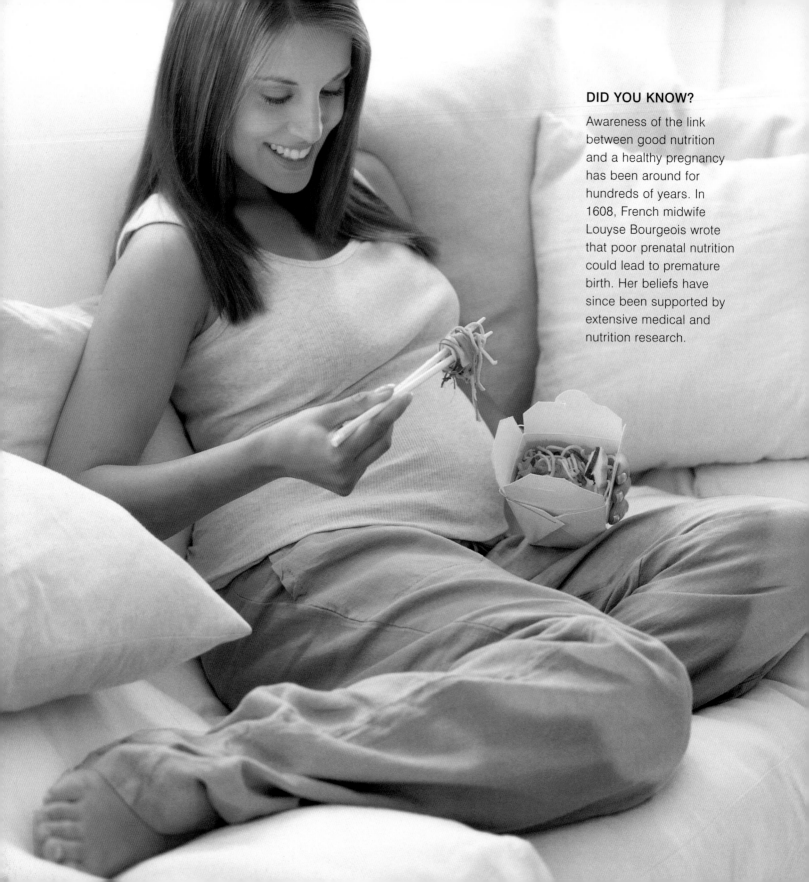

DID YOU KNOW?

Awareness of the link between good nutrition and a healthy pregnancy has been around for hundreds of years. In 1608, French midwife Louyse Bourgeois wrote that poor prenatal nutrition could lead to premature birth. Her beliefs have since been supported by extensive medical and nutrition research.

How to assess your pre-pregnancy weight

The Body Mass Index (BMI) is the internationally accepted way of finding out how healthy your weight is. Use this chart as a guide, and discuss any weight concerns with your doctor. Please remember that this chart is definitely not for use during pregnancy.

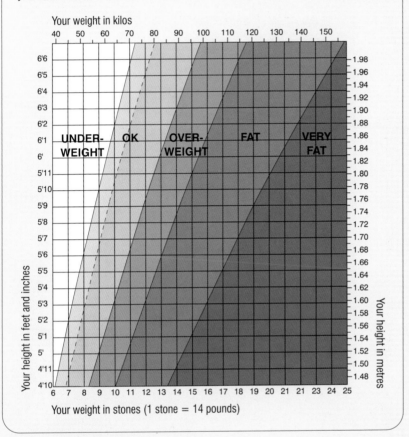

Your weight in kilos

UNDER-WEIGHT   OK   OVER-WEIGHT   FAT   VERY FAT

Your height in feet and inches

Your height in metres

Your weight in stones (1 stone = 14 pounds)

FATHERS-TO-BE

The health of the father-to-be is also important for a successful pregnancy. Poor diet, too much alcohol, smoking, and recreational drugs influence the health, production, and movement of sperm. Being overweight has also been linked to reduced fertility, according to research from the American National Institute of Environmental Health Sciences. When it comes to diet, key nutrients involved in the production of healthy sperm include zinc, selenium, folic acid, vitamin C, and omega-3 and omega-6 fatty acids (*see* page 17). Eating at least five portions daily of antioxidant-rich fruit and vegetables has been associated with having more active sperm.

PLANNING A BABY CHECKLIST

Both parents-to-be will benefit from most of these.

- ❍ Enjoy a healthy balanced diet.
- ❍ Aim to avoid alcohol.
- ❍ If you smoke, work to stop.
- ❍ Aim to be a healthy weight.
- ❍ Check any medications, ointments, herbal remedies, or nutritional supplements.
- ❍ Take a 400-microgram (mcg) supplement of folic acid daily (mother only).
- ❍ Follow food hygiene and food safety advice.
- ❍ Enjoy regular physical activity.
- ❍ See your doctor about any existing health problems.

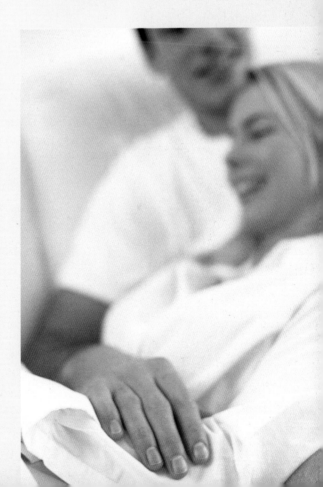

While you are pregnant

Food is fuel. It provides the energy and nutrients you need for every bodily function and activity—breathing, digestion, brain, nerve, and muscle function, heartbeats, hormone production, temperature regulation, immunity, movement, and exercise—as well as supporting the healthy growth and development of your baby.

Food is made up of carbohydrates, fats, protein, fiber, vitamins, minerals, and water. Plant foods also provide a wide range of beneficial compounds called "phytochemicals," and many work as protective antioxidants (see page 13). Energy in food is measured in calories and is provided by fats, carbohydrates (sugars and starches), and protein. Vitamins and minerals are needed in relatively tiny amounts, but are essential for growth and development and to regulate the body's chemical processes and functions. Some minerals also have a structural role, for example calcium in bones and teeth. From the placenta, through the umbilical cord, your developing baby will absorb these vital nutrients—from the stores you already have in your body, and from what is supplied in your diet. Your body also becomes more efficient at absorbing key nutrients to help ensure your baby gets what it needs.

CHOOSING A HEALTHY BALANCED DIET

Eating well during pregnancy gives your baby a wonderful start in life. There is no need to follow a special diet. Apart from taking more care with food safety (see page 28), the guidelines for a healthy diet are much the same as at any other time of your life. You can get an optimal diet packed with over 50 vital nutrients by choosing a variety of foods from each of the different groups each day in healthy proportions (see Eating for Good Health diagram below).

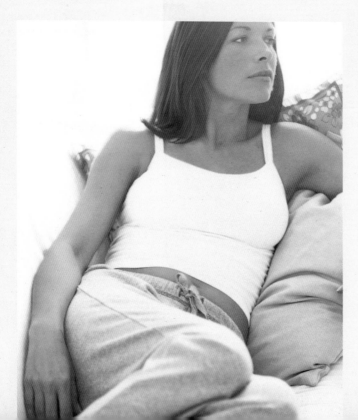

EATING FOR GOOD HEALTH

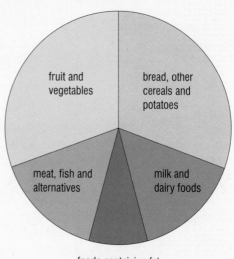

fruit and vegetables

bread, other cereals and potatoes

meat, fish and alternatives

milk and dairy foods

foods containing fat
foods containing sugar

These food groups are:

○ Healthy energy foods such as whole-grain bread, pasta, rice, potatoes, cereals, and noodles. Make them a base for your meals and include slow energy release whole-grain types for extra B vitamins, minerals, and fiber.

○ At least five portions of fruit and vegetables—fresh, frozen, canned, dried, and juiced all count. They brim with folic acid, vitamin C, beta-carotene, magnesium, potassium, fiber, and protective antioxidants.

○ Three servings of milk and dairy products (or calcium-fortified soy alternatives) for protein, calcium, zinc, and B vitamins. A serving could be 1 cup milk, 6 ounces yogurt, or 1 ounce hard cheese. Low-fat milk and yogurt are just as rich in calcium as full-fat varieties.

○ Two to three moderate servings of lean meat, fish, chicken, eggs, pulses, tofu, nuts and seeds for protein, iron, B vitamins, zinc, magnesium, and selenium.

○ Modest amounts of unsaturated oils and spreads for vitamins D and E and essential fats. Keep to small amounts of fatty, sugary, and salty foods.

What about drinks?

As your body changes and baby grows, your fluid requirements increase. Aim to drink 8 cups or glasses a day—more if it is hot or you are exercising. Water is ideal as a main drink but milk, smoothies, juices, infusions (*see* page 134), and some tea or coffee (*see* page 29) also count. If your urine is a light straw color, you are drinking enough, but if it is dark and in small volumes, you need more. If you find your urine is dark yellow after you take your prenatal vitamin, do not worry. This is likely due to the riboflavin in the vitamin and not dehydration.

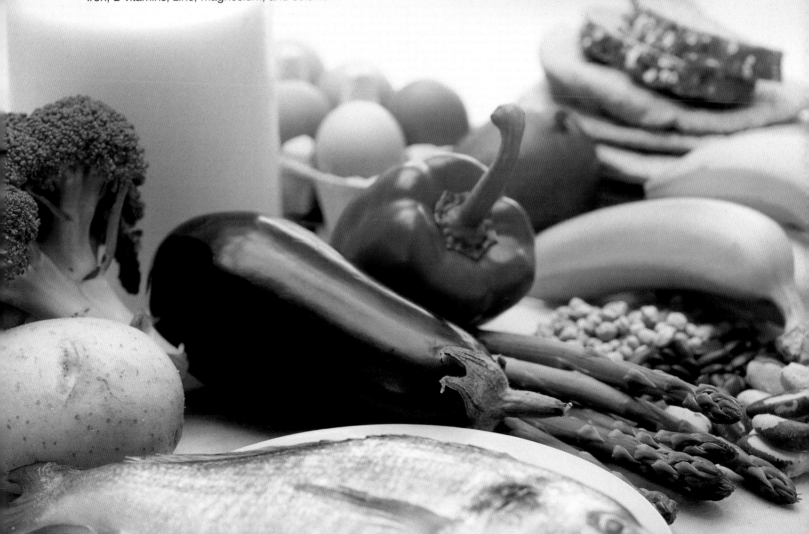

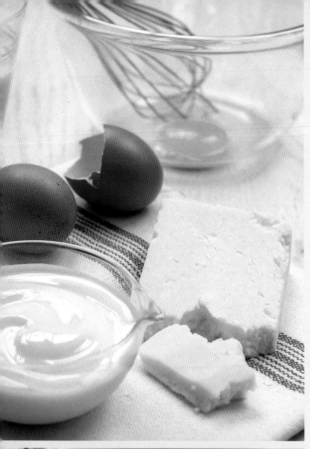

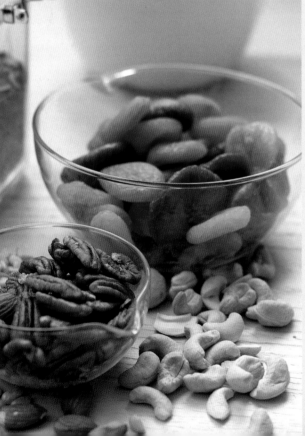

Key nutrients during pregnancy

All essential nutrients have a crucial role to play in promoting the growth and development of a healthy baby. On the following pages are the nutrients that are most important for both mother and baby.

PROTEIN

Protein is vital for the growth and repair of body tissues—including your developing baby's new cells and organs—as well as the production of hormones and other chemical messengers that regulate body processes. Your protein intake needs to be increased by a small amount during pregnancy. This can easily be covered with a balanced diet, and most American women will actually find they get enough protein to cover the needs of pregnancy.

Good sources include:

❍ All types of meat, poultry, fish, eggs, dairy foods, legumes, tofu, nuts, seeds

IRON

Iron is needed to help make new cells, including red blood cells. It is vital not just for your baby (who will take what he/she needs even if it means you go short), but also to support the increase in red blood cells in your body as your pregnancy progresses. Your body cleverly adapts by nearly tripling how much iron it absorbs, and you no longer lose blood from monthly periods, so overall dietary iron needs don't increase. But you still need to ensure a good intake to prevent iron deficiency, which can make you tired and increase the risk of premature delivery. Iron is best absorbed from red meat, chicken, and fish, but you can boost absorption from other foods by eating vitamin C-rich plant foods at the same meal (see page 16).

Good sources include:

❍ Red meat and poultry—especially the dark meat

❍ Shrimp, mussels and oily fish such as mackerel, sardines, canned pilchards,

❍ Legumes, peas, beans, lentils

❍ Iron-fortified breakfast cereals, whole-wheat bread, quinoa

❍ Dark green leafy vegetables such as watercress, spinach, kale, spring greens, arugula

❍ Dried fruit—figs and apricots

CALCIUM

Calcium helps maintain healthy bones and teeth. It is also needed for nerve and muscle function, and blood clotting. Your developing baby is very good at taking what it needs, so if your diet is short of calcium, your bones will supply it. Your calcium needs don't actually increase during pregnancy, as you absorb it more efficiently (as long as you have enough vitamin D, *see* pages 16–17) and pass less out in your urine.

Good sources include:

- Milk, yogurt, cheese
- Calcium-fortified soy milk, soy yogurt, tofu, orange juice
- Fish with edible small bones—canned sardines, pilchards, salmon, and fresh whitebait
- Dried figs
- Baked beans, chickpeas
- Almonds, tahini (sesame seed) paste
- Dark green leafy vegetables such as watercress, kale, spring greens, bok choy, broccoli (but not spinach)
- Bread, Swiss-style muesli

MAGNESIUM

Magnesium helps your body use energy from food, and together with calcium plays a role in nerve transmission and muscle movement. It also gives hardness and rigidity to bones, and is needed to build new body cells.

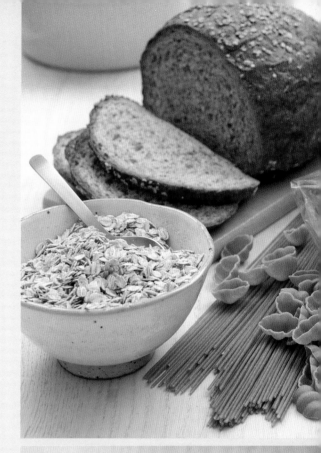

Good sources include:

- All types of fish and shellfish
- All types of nuts and seeds
- Green leafy vegetables
- All types of beans
- Whole-grain breads and cereals

ZINC

Zinc is essential for cell division, so is especially crucial in the early stages of pregnancy (in the 10th week, the one cell that we all start life as multiplies into 10 billion cells!). It also keeps your immune system healthy. You won't need to alter your diet to include extra zinc, as your body absorbs it more effectively during pregnancy.

Good sources include:

- Beef, lamb, pork, chicken
- Oysters (cooked), canned crab, canned sardines
- Pumpkin seeds, cashews, pecans, pine nuts
- Milk, dairy foods
- Legumes
- Oats, wheatgerm, whole-grain breads and cereals, quinoa

FOLATE OR FOLIC ACID

Folic acid is a B vitamin (folate is the form found naturally in food) that helps make red blood cells and is essential for cell division. In the early weeks of pregnancy, it plays a key role in the normal development of your baby's spinal cord, referred

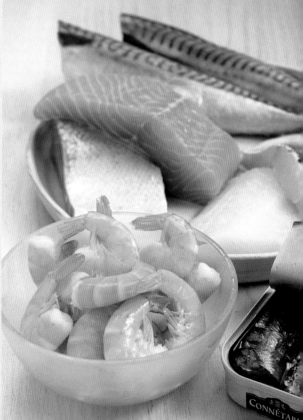

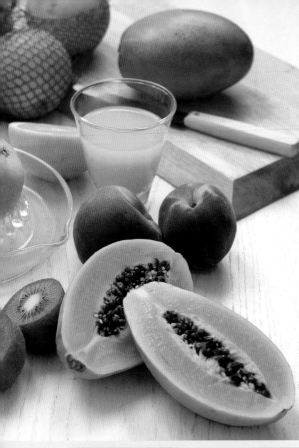

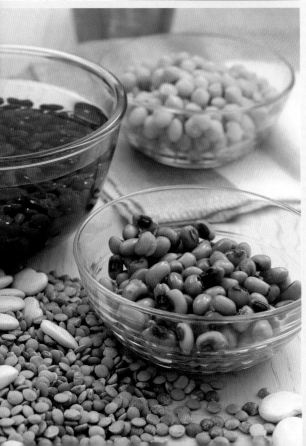

to as "the neural tube." If it doesn't develop normally, a baby can be born with neural-tube defects such as spina bifida. Rather than rely on diet alone, research has shown the importance of taking a 400-mcg supplement of folic acid daily (*see* page 8), as well as eating folic acid-rich foods, to reduce the risk of neural-tube defects.

Good sources include:

○ Dark green leafy vegetables, including lettuce, Brussels sprouts

○ Black-eyed peas, chickpeas

○ Fortified breakfast cereals and bread

○ Orange juice

○ Asparagus, beets (not pickled), okra, parsnips, potatoes, blackberries

○ Tahini (sesame seed) paste, cashews

VITAMIN A

Your vitamin A requirements increase during pregnancy. It is needed to build new cells and tissues, and supports the development of your baby's immune system (as well as keeping yours in good working order). Retinol, found in animal foods, is one form of vitamin A. Beta-carotene, found in plant foods, is converted inside our bodies into vitamin A. While we need some in our diet, extremely high intakes of retinol can be harmful to developing babies,

so rich sources such as liver should be avoided, and care should also be taken with supplements (*see* page 21).

Good sources include:

○ Retinol—eggs, cheese, kidney, butter, margarine

○ Beta-carotene—red, orange, and dark green leafy vegetables and fruit such as carrots, bell peppers, apricots, mangoes, sweet potatoes, kale, spinach, watercress

VITAMIN C

Vitamin C is needed to help build your developing baby's tissues, bones, and blood vessels, so your requirement increases during pregnancy. It also boosts iron absorption from non-meat foods, is a powerful antioxidant that helps to protect cells from damage, and supports the immune system.

Good sources include:

○ Fruit and vegetable juices

○ Citrus fruit, berries, black currants, melon, kiwi fruit, papaya

○ Bell peppers, broccoli, green leafy vegetables, cabbage, potatoes, tomatoes

VITAMIN D

Vitamin D is essential for the proper absorption and use of calcium in the body, and for the normal development of your baby's bones and teeth. It also helps build a strong immune system. Few foods contain vitamin D, and our major supply is from the action of some gentle summer sunlight on the skin. Once made, it is stored in the liver for use during the winter. To ensure needs are met, doctors recommend that all pregnant women should take a daily 5-mcg vitamin D supplement (see page 21). This is particularly important for women who rarely go outdoors, always cover their skin when outside, or are of Asian or African origin.

Good sources include:

- Oily fish
- Eggs
- Fortified foods e.g. breakfast cereals, soy milks, and spreads
- Hard cheese e.g. cheddar
- Butter, margarine

OMEGA-3 FATTY ACIDS

Omega-3s are essential for building healthy linings for every cell in the body. They also help regulate functions such as inflammation, immunity, and childbirth contractions. We generally get enough omega-6 fatty acids in our diets but it is important to pay attention to omega-3s. Certain types called "long-chain omega-3 fatty acids" (also referred to as EPA and DHA) are vital during pregnancy for babies' eye, nerve, and brain development, as well as

maintaining the health of the nervous system later in life. Oily fish are the best source of long-chain omega-3s. Pregnant women should eat no more than two portions a week (see page 29). Our body can also make small amounts from alpha-linolenic acid, the omega-3 found in plant foods.

Good sources include:

Long-chain omega-3s (EPA/DHA)

- Oily fish such as salmon, sardines, mackerel, pilchards, trout, tuna
- Crab, shrimp
- Omega-3-enriched eggs (some are suitable for vegetarians)

Plant sources of omega-3 (alpha-linolenic acid)—important for vegetarians (see page 19)

- Canola oil, walnut oil, soy oil
- Flaxseed, pumpkin seeds, walnuts
- Tofu, wheat germ
- Dark green leafy vegetables such as watercress, spinach, mâche, mint

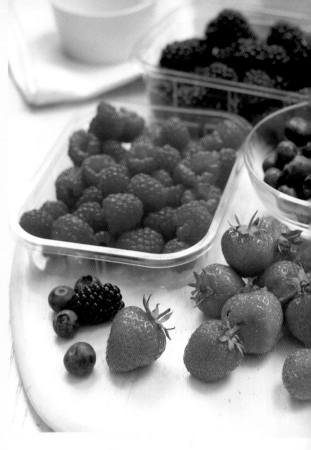

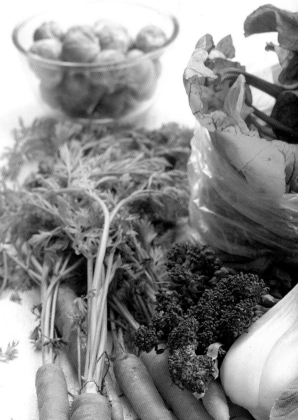

Omega-3 and baby

Your baby's brain and nervous system has a growth spurt during the last 12 weeks of your pregnancy, making a good intake of omega-3 fatty acids especially important then.

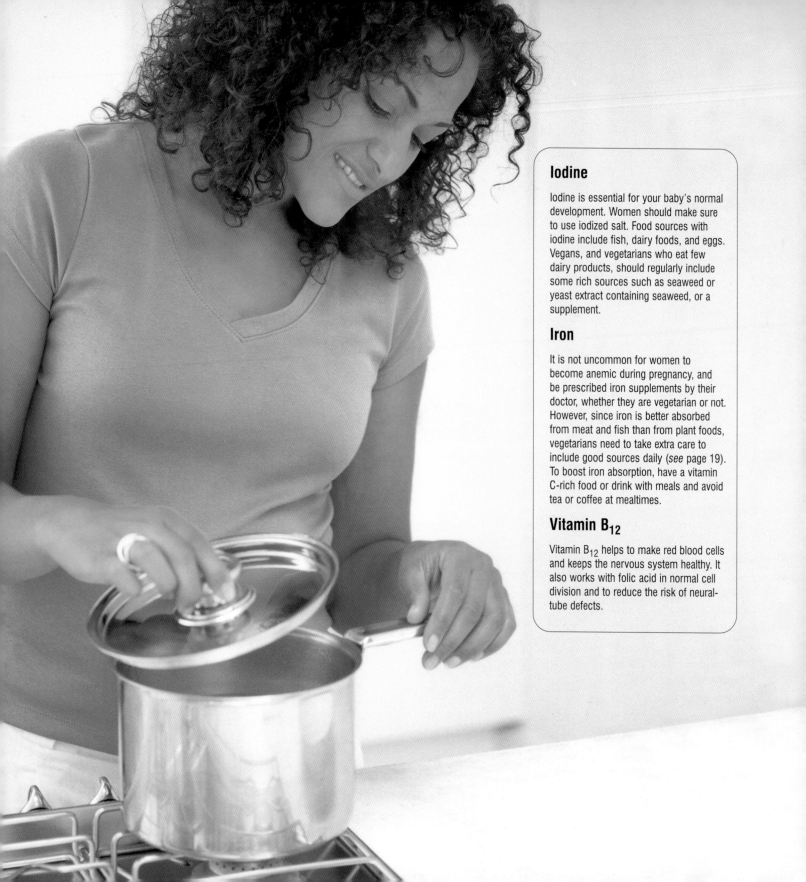

Iodine

Iodine is essential for your baby's normal development. Women should make sure to use iodized salt. Food sources with iodine include fish, dairy foods, and eggs. Vegans, and vegetarians who eat few dairy products, should regularly include some rich sources such as seaweed or yeast extract containing seaweed, or a supplement.

Iron

It is not uncommon for women to become anemic during pregnancy, and be prescribed iron supplements by their doctor, whether they are vegetarian or not. However, since iron is better absorbed from meat and fish than from plant foods, vegetarians need to take extra care to include good sources daily (*see* page 19). To boost iron absorption, have a vitamin C-rich food or drink with meals and avoid tea or coffee at mealtimes.

Vitamin B_{12}

Vitamin B_{12} helps to make red blood cells and keeps the nervous system healthy. It also works with folic acid in normal cell division and to reduce the risk of neural-tube defects.

IF YOU ARE VEGETARIAN

There is no reason why a vegetarian or vegan diet can't be followed during pregnancy. But, in addition to general balanced diet guidelines, some areas need special attention.

If you are vegetarian (eat eggs and dairy foods but no meat or fish):

- Include some eggs, legumes (peas, beans, or lentils), nuts, seeds, or tofu, two or three times a day, for protein, iron, and zinc.
- Include three servings of dairy foods daily for protein, calcium, and B vitamins (*see* pages 14–17).
- Enjoy a variety of fruit, vegetables, whole-grain breads and cereals, pasta, rice, and noodles.
- Include vegetarian foods containing omega-3 fatty acids daily (*see* page 17).
- Follow the guidance for folic acid and vitamin D supplements (*see* pages 15–16).

If you are vegan (do not eat eggs, dairy foods, meat or fish):

- For protein, iron, and zinc, include some legumes (peas, beans, or lentils), nuts, seeds, or tofu, two or three times a day.
- Enjoy a variety of fruit, vegetables, whole-grain breads and cereals, grains, pasta, rice, and noodles.
- Include three servings of calcium-fortified soy milk or yogurt and include other non-dairy sources of calcium (*see* page 15).
- Include plant foods containing omega-3 fatty acid sources daily (*see* page 17) and good sources of iodine (*see* fact box on page 18).
- Follow the guidance regarding folic acid and vitamin D supplements. Vitamin B_{12} is only found naturally in meat, fish, dairy foods, and eggs, so a daily supplement or B_{12}-fortified foods is advisable.

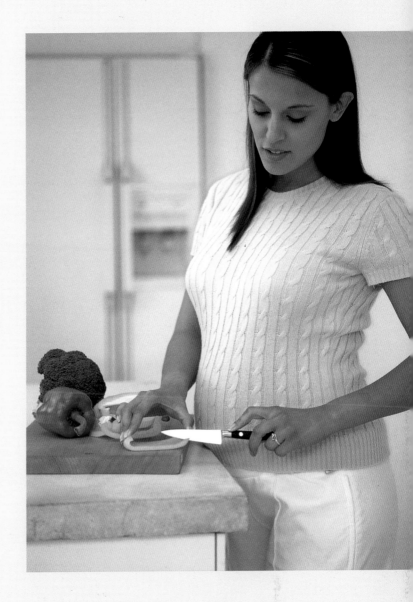

IF YOU FOLLOW A SPECIAL DIET

This book provides general information about diet and pregnancy, with a range of recipes containing different ingredients. If you have a food intolerance or medical condition that requires a special or restricted diet, then do talk to your doctor and registered dietitian to ensure your diet is tailored to meet your nutritional needs during pregnancy.

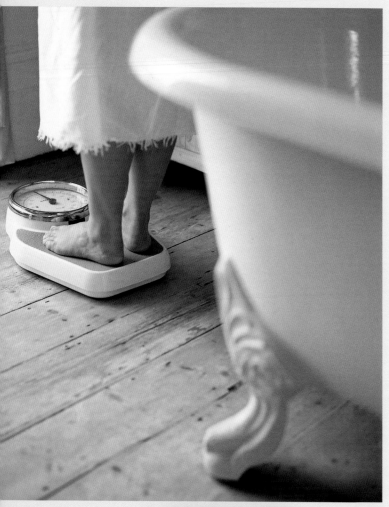

WEIGHT GAIN

It is essential for a healthy pregnancy to gain weight as your baby grows and develops. As well as the weight of your baby, there is the placenta, breast enlargement, extra blood and fluids, and additional fat stores to consider. Different women will gain different amounts of weight, but a healthy range for women who were a healthy weight before becoming pregnant seems to be about 25 to 35 lb over the whole of their pregnancy.

Gaining too much weight increases your risk of high blood pressure, gestational diabetes, and labor complications—and of staying overweight after your baby is born. It may also increase your baby's risk of being overweight as a toddler. If you are overweight when you learn you are pregnant, it is important not to try to lose weight. Instead, eat wisely, think twice about fatty and sugary foods and drinks, and ideally aim for a weight gain of between 15 and 25 lb.

Eating well is also important if you are underweight at the beginning of your pregnancy. Aim for a weight gain of between 28 and 40 lb, to help ensure your baby reaches a healthy birth weight (*see* page 9). These are guidelines only, so do talk to your doctor, dietitian, or midwife if you are concerned about any aspect of your weight.

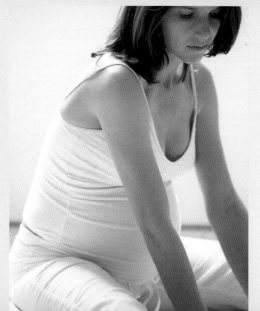

Quality not quantity

Being pregnant doesn't mean eating for two. Simply enjoy regular meals and some planned nutritious snacks, and focus on the quality of your diet. You will also find that your appetite fluctuates throughout your pregnancy. Your calorie needs only increase during the last six months of pregnancy, and then by about 300 calories a day, while requirements for protein and vitamins A, B_1, B_2, C, D, and folic acid increase slightly throughout. One simple way to meet these extra needs is by snacking on fruit, whole-grain breads or cereals, and milk or soymilk. Plus there are plenty of nutritious recipes and snack ideas in this book.

HAVING MORE THAN ONE BABY?

If you are expecting more than one baby, not surprisingly your nutritional needs and healthy level of weight gain will be higher. If you are expecting twins, US recommendations are to have an additional 450 calories daily (from nutritious foods) and gain between 35 and 45 lb overall. Gaining a good amount of weight between 20 and 24 weeks of pregnancy will increase both babies' chances of being born with healthy birth weights. To help support the growth and development of your babies, a prenatal vitamin and mineral supplement (*see* page 8 and below) is also advisable. Getting enough rest and having more regular antenatal check-ups are also vital, so do seek individual advice from your midwife and doctor.

WHAT ABOUT SUPPLEMENTS?

All women are advised to take 400 mcg folic acid per day if they are trying to conceive. This should be taken until the 12th week of pregnancy to reduce the risk of neural tube defects such as spina bifida. They are also advised to take 5 mcg vitamin D daily. You may prefer to take these individually or as part of a prenatal supplement, which is specially designed for women planning pregnancy and who are pregnant, and contains a range of vitamins and minerals. While not essential if you are eating a balanced diet, some women like to take them as an insurance policy. They can be particularly helpful for women having more than one baby, teenage mothers-to-be (who are still growing themselves), vegans (who should ensure they have an adequate vitamin B_{12} and iodine intake), and women who have a poor diet (sometimes due to lengthy morning sickness). Remember that too much vitamin A can be harmful to your baby, and this is in fish liver oil supplements as well as various vitamin supplements. Always check the suitability of any supplements with your doctor, pharmacist, or midwife.

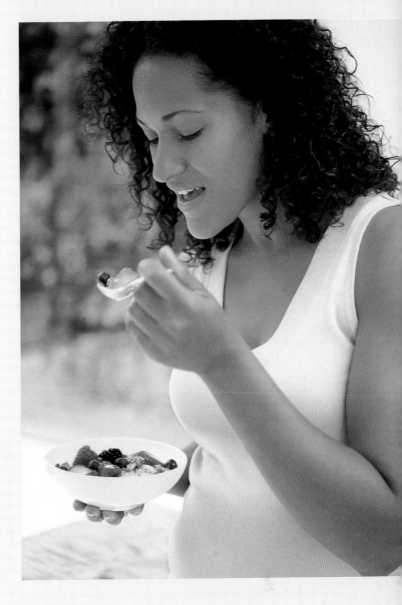

Your weight

During the first trimester of pregnancy, you gain about 3 lb just from the extra amount of blood in your body. Sometimes gaining a lot of weight quite quickly is due to fluid retention. If this happens, consult your doctor or midwife before you limit how much you are eating.

Common upsets during pregnancy

During pregnancy, many changes will be happening in your body. With these changes can come physical upsets, which affect each woman differently. Some experience many symptoms, while others only have a few or none at all. Some upsets continue for several weeks or months, and others only last for a short period of time.

MORNING SICKNESS

Morning sickness, which in reality can occur at any time of day, is a common part of pregnancy, affecting around 7 in 10 women with varying intensity. There is no clear cause, but changing hormone levels are thought to be the most likely culprit. It typically starts between 6 and 7 weeks of pregnancy and usually resolves by 12 to 14 weeks. Extreme tiredness is also common, and is probably nature's way of saying "slow down a bit." One good thing is that it's linked to a reduced risk of miscarriage. Don't worry if you aren't eating very much for a little while. Just do the best you can. Most likely, you will have plenty of stored energy and nutrients for your baby to make use of.

WHAT HELPS

Nausea is worse when you haven't eaten for many hours, meaning an empty stomach and dwindling blood sugar levels.

○ Eat small, light frequent meals and snacks. Try to have breakfast —a fruit smoothie, toast, or small bowl of cereal may help.

○ Keep plain or ginger cookies, or crackers, by your bed and eat some before getting up in the morning or if you wake in the night. Get up slowly in the morning.

○ Rest and relax as much as you can. Feeling tired or anxious can make nausea worse.

○ If the smell of cooking upsets you, cold foods can be more manageable e.g. a chilled soup, granola bars or rice cakes, cold frittata, potato or pasta salad, melon, yogurt, or ice cream.

○ Air rooms well, and try to avoid smells that upset you.

○ When you feel sick, try ginger infusions or ginger ale, or sucking on sweets or a popsicle.

○ If you feel so sick you can't drink or keep food down, or also have a high fever, then contact your doctor or healthcare professional.

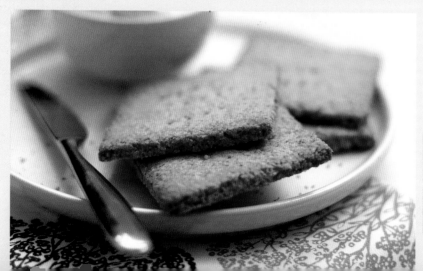

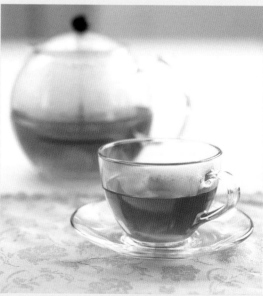

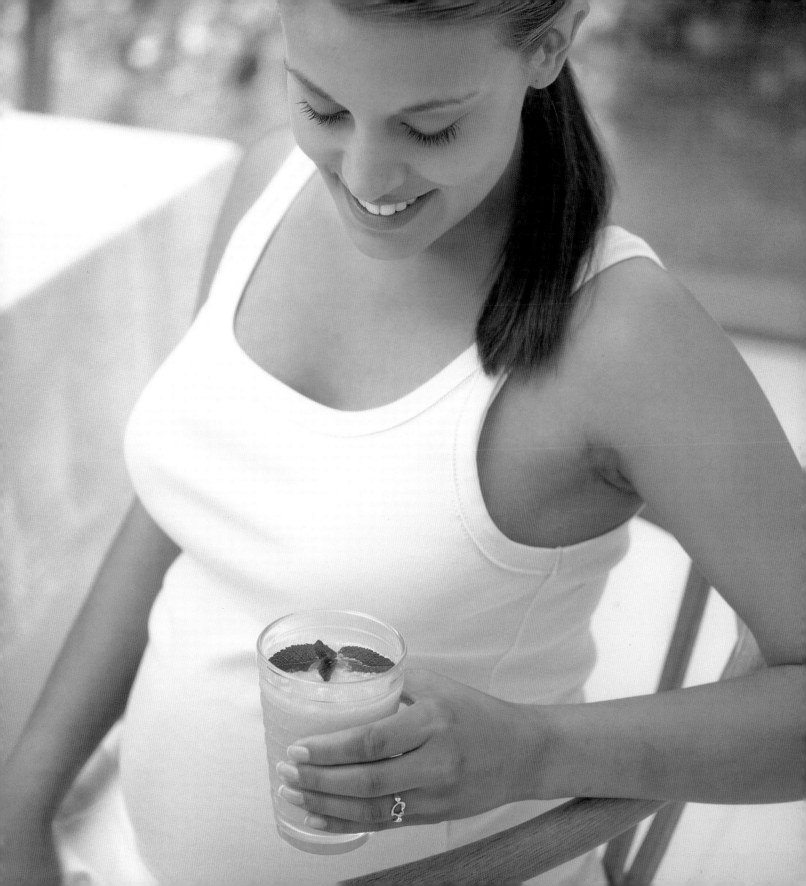

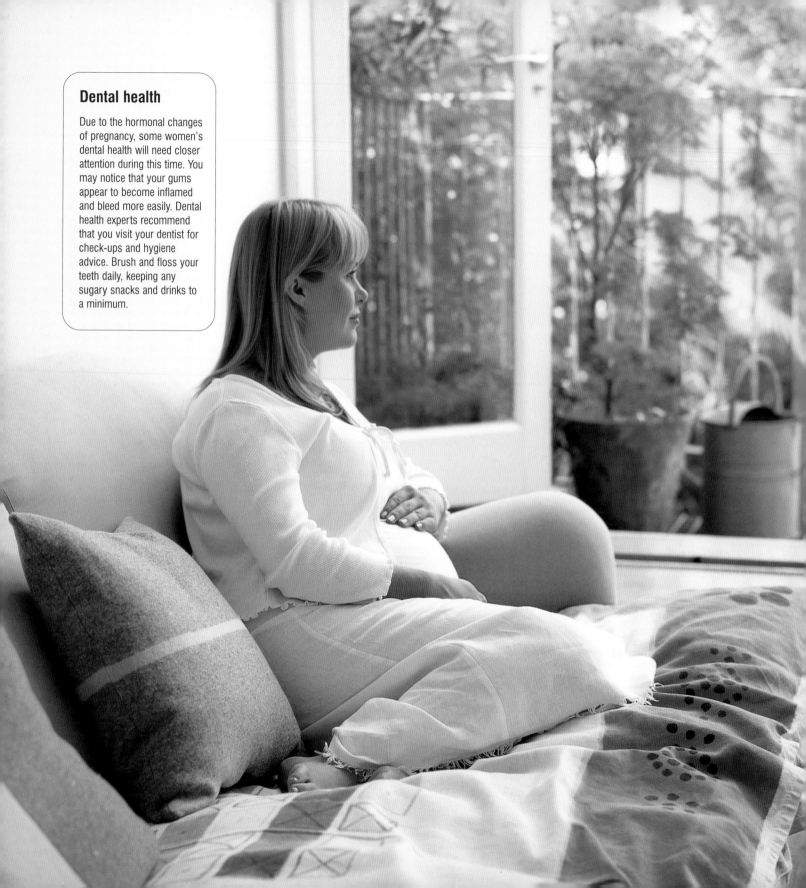

Dental health

Due to the hormonal changes of pregnancy, some women's dental health will need closer attention during this time. You may notice that your gums appear to become inflamed and bleed more easily. Dental health experts recommend that you visit your dentist for check-ups and hygiene advice. Brush and floss your teeth daily, keeping any sugary snacks and drinks to a minimum.

FOOD CRAVINGS

Pregnancy is notorious for food cravings and food aversions. Their cause isn't clear, but the strongest theory relates to higher levels of hormones such as estrogen. Then there's the comfort factor of foods that help women deal with the tiredness, nausea, taste changes, bloating, or mood swings these hormones can cause. This might explain the cravings for ice cream, chocolate, and childhood favorites—but cravings for pickles and weird combinations remain a mystery! You need to enjoy food as well as stay healthy, so the main advice is to be aware of your food cravings or aversions, then take action if they put you at risk of an unbalanced diet, excess weight gain (or loss), or eating unsafe foods.

HEARTBURN

Heartburn is common during pregnancy. Higher levels of the hormone progesterone relax the valve between the stomach and esophagus (food pipe), making it easier for stomach acid to rise up, irritating the esophagus, and causing a burning sensation in the middle of the chest. It's usually worse in the later stages of pregnancy when your growing baby naturally pushes against your stomach. Heartburn usually disappears following childbirth.

If you suffer from heartburn, try the following:

❍ Eat five or six small meals over the day, not three large ones.

❍ Spread drinks over the day too, and avoid drinking large quantities at meals.

❍ Avoid fried or rich foods, or any items that make it worse. Common culprits are carbonated drinks, orange juice, pickles, peppermint, and chocolate.

❍ Don't lie down or bend over directly after eating.

❍ Keep the head of your bed higher than the foot of your bed, or place pillows under your shoulders to help prevent stomach acids from rising into your esophagus.

❍ Wear loose-fitting clothing.

❍ If heartburn persists, see your doctor. They can prescribe medications that are safe to take during pregnancy.

CONSTIPATION

High levels of pregnancy hormones such as progesterone also have a relaxing effect on the muscles that make the bowel contract. This means the bowel can be sluggish, making you prone to constipation. Prescribed iron supplements can also cause constipation. Here are some tips for preventing and managing it.

❍ Include fiber-rich foods at every meal. Choose from whole-grain bread and crackers, whole-grain or bran-based breakfast cereals, brown rice, legumes, vegetables, fresh and dried fruit, nuts or seeds.

❍ Drink plenty of water and other fluids (*see* page 13) each day.

❍ Try a daily probiotic drink or yogurt.

❍ Enjoy a daily walk or other suitable exercise (*see* page 34).

❍ Avoid putting off the urge to use the toilet.

❍ If constipation persists, talk to your doctor or midwife. They may recommend a safe laxative.

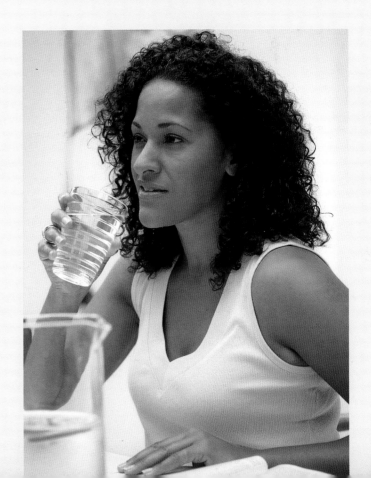

Making safe food choices

If you find the whole issue of what is or isn't safe to eat and drink confusing, you aren't alone. Conflicting advice, newspaper headlines, and your in-built desire to do the best thing can often make deciding what to buy and consume a bit frustrating. But there are clear guidelines. Armed with this knowledge and your own common sense, you will soon be confident about the risky items to skip, and able to enjoy a tasty and nutritious diet.

LIVER AND VITAMIN A

Foods and supplements with high levels of vitamin A (retinol) should be avoided. We all need some vitamin A for good health, but no more than 5000 IU is recommended due to its link to birth defects. Supplements containing retinol, including fish liver oils, should be avoided unless they have been recommended and approved by your doctor, pharmacist, or other healthcare professional. The plant form of vitamin A, known as beta-carotene (found in orange, red, yellow, and dark green vegetables and fruit) is safe.

Inform your doctor if you have been using Accutane or Retin-A for acne and wrinkle treatment. These forms of vitamin A are not recommended during pregnancy due to their increased risk of birth defects.

FOOD SAFETY

All of us should take care with food hygiene and make safe choices to avoid food poisoning. This becomes especially important when you are pregnant, as your immune system works less effectively, making you more vulnerable to serious infections from potentially harmful bacteria or parasites. These infections may not only make you ill, but could harm your developing baby. This may sound worrying, but the risk of getting one of these infections is actually very low. If you follow the food safety advice, you can easily keep food hazards at bay.

Safety with pets

- Always wash your hands after handling pets.

- Wear rubber gloves when handling pet litter trays.

- Keep pets off surfaces where you prepare food, and ideally out of the kitchen.

- Wear rubber gloves when gardening (to avoid contamination from soil fouled by cats).

Quick reference guide to foods to eat or avoid

RISKY FOOD-BORNE BACTERIA/PARASITES	WHAT TO AVOID	WHAT YOU CAN EAT
Listeria can cause mild flu-like symptoms. Could lead to miscarriage, stillbirth, or severe illness in newborns. Rare, and risk is extremely small.	• Blue-veined cheeses • Soft mold-ripened cheeses (e.g. Camembert, Brie) • Soft, unpasteurized goat or sheep cheese • Fresh pâté—any type, including fish or vegetable • Chilled prepared meals that are not thoroughly heated	• Hard cheeses (e.g. cheddar, Edam, halloumi, Parmesan) • Cream cheese, cottage cheese, cheese spread, ricotta, yogurt • Canned pâté if labeled 'pasteurized' (not liver pâté) • Piping hot prepared meals that are fully heated through
Salmonella infection affects the mother only (severe vomiting and diarrhea), but her fever can affect the baby.	• Raw or partially cooked eggs • Homemade or restaurant mayonnaise, sauces, ice cream, or mousse made with raw egg • Raw or undercooked poultry or meat • Unpasteurized fruit juices	• Eggs cooked until white and yolk are solid • Storebought mayonnaise, ice cream, mousses, or any made with pasteurized egg • Thoroughly cooked poultry or meat. No pink meat; juices should run clear
Toxoplasmosis is caused by a parasite found in animal droppings, soil, and undercooked meat. It can cause mild flu-like symptoms, but sometimes none at all. It can cause brain and eye damage in the baby. Extremely rare.	• Raw or undercooked meat, including cured meat (e.g. salami, prosciutto) • Unpasteurized goat milk • Unwashed vegetables and salads • Take care with contact with pets (*see* fact box on page 26)	• Thoroughly cooked poultry or meat (and always wash hands thoroughly after handling raw meat) • Pasteurized or UHT goat milk • Washed vegetables and salads, including washed bagged salads
Other bacteria can cause unpleasant food poisoning, e.g. campylobacter.	• Raw or undercooked shellfish • Unpasteurized cow, goat, or sheep milk as well as yogurt made from it • Unwashed fruit and vegetables	• Pasteurized milk of any type and yogurt made from it • Thoroughly cooked shellfish (e.g. shrimp, mussels, oysters) • Washed fruit and vegetables

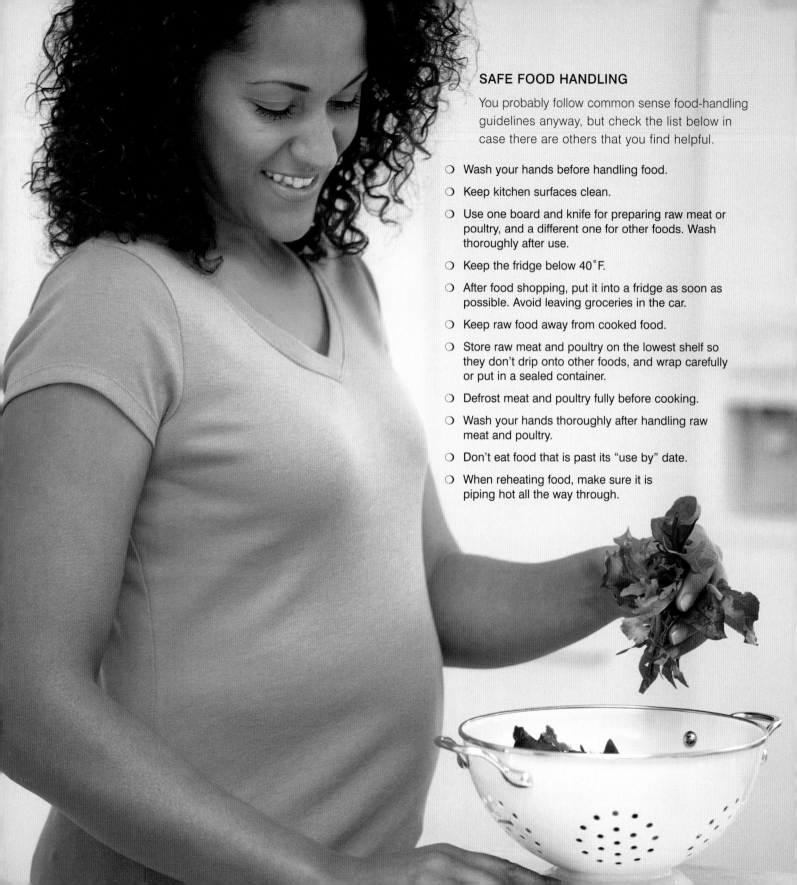

SAFE FOOD HANDLING

You probably follow common sense food-handling guidelines anyway, but check the list below in case there are others that you find helpful.

❍ Wash your hands before handling food.

❍ Keep kitchen surfaces clean.

❍ Use one board and knife for preparing raw meat or poultry, and a different one for other foods. Wash thoroughly after use.

❍ Keep the fridge below 40˚F.

❍ After food shopping, put it into a fridge as soon as possible. Avoid leaving groceries in the car.

❍ Keep raw food away from cooked food.

❍ Store raw meat and poultry on the lowest shelf so they don't drip onto other foods, and wrap carefully or put in a sealed container.

❍ Defrost meat and poultry fully before cooking.

❍ Wash your hands thoroughly after handling raw meat and poultry.

❍ Don't eat food that is past its "use by" date.

❍ When reheating food, make sure it is piping hot all the way through.

WHAT ABOUT FISH AND SHELLFISH?

Fish provides nutrients such as iron, protein, magnesium, iodine, selenium, B vitamins, long-chain omega-3 fatty acids, and vitamin D. However, some fish contain pollutants such as mercury, dioxins, and PCBs (polychlorinated biphenyls). Pregnant women are advised to eat less than 12 ounces fish per week:

❍ Consume no more than 6 ounces "albacore" or "white" tuna or tuna steak each week.

❍ Fish is a good source of protein but swordfish, shark, king mackerel, and tilefish should be avoided due to their levels of methyl mercury. Pregnant women can enjoy other types of fish such as shrimp and salmon but limit their intake to 12 ounces a week.

Fish—how to tell your white from your oily

Fish is very nutritious and great to include in your weekly diet while you are pregnant. Compared to white fish, oily fish has a higher content of beneficial long-chain omega-3 fatty acids (see page 17). Use this guide to help you, taking care to follow the above limits on how much to eat of certain fish during pregnancy.

Oily fish

Salmon, sardines, trout, fresh tuna, blue fish, kippers, herrings, anchovies, whitebait, sprats, and eel.

White or non-oily fish

Cod, haddock, pollock, plaice, canned light tuna, sole, flounder, halibut, sea bass, ocean perch, rockfish, red snapper, and monkfish.

CAFFEINE—IS IT SAFE?

Caffeine occurs naturally in a range of foods, such as coffee, tea (including green tea), and chocolate. It's also added to soft drinks and "energy" drinks, and cold and flu remedies (always check medications with your doctor).

High intakes of caffeine have been associated with an increased risk of low birth weight or miscarriage, so you should limit the amount you have each day. The American College of Obstetricians and Gynecologists recommend that pregnant women limit consumption to the caffeine equivalent of 1 to 2 cups of coffee per day. Use of caffeine during pregnancy should be discussed with your healthcare professional or doctor.

IS IT SAFE TO CONSUME ARTIFICIAL SWEETENERS DURING PREGNANCY?

Low-calorie (artificial) sweeteners can be used by pregnant women who have diabetes or by those who need to control caloric intake. Since restricting calories is not necessary for most pregnancies, many experts recommend avoiding low-calorie sweeteners. As research on this matter is controversial, you should discuss this with your healthcare professional or doctor if you do not wish to avoid low-calorie sweeteners.

ALCOHOL—THE BOTTOM LINE

Women who are pregnant or planning to become pregnant are advised not to drink alcohol. Alcohol passes from the bloodstream and through the placenta and can harm the developing baby.

Once baby is born

Congratulations! Now that your baby has joined you in the outside world, continue to take care of yourself, as well as them, to give you the energy you need at this exciting, busy, and often tiring time. If you are breastfeeding, your body requires energy and fluid to produce the milk your rapidly growing baby needs, and to help you combat tiredness. On average, breastfeeding women need more calories daily and a nutrient-rich diet. Many women decide to continue to take a multivitamin, but a well-nourished woman with a healthy diet does not need routine vitamin or mineral supplementation. You should find that your appetite and thirst naturally increase to help you achieve that. Some of those calories will come from the fat stores you laid down during pregnancy. Meanwhile, keep up your balanced diet with regular meals and snacks and slow energy release foods, aiming to have three to four servings of dairy foods, which also boost vitamin and mineral intake, a day. This is largely to replenish and maintain your nutritional needs. If necessary, your body draws on its own nutrient stores (including your bone calcium, which is restored after weaning).

Make sure you drink at least 8 glasses or cups of water and suitable drinks (see page 13) a day. Have a drink such as water, diluted juice, or low-fat milk within easy reach when you are breastfeeding, as this is a time when women can feel quite thirsty. Drinking plenty of fluids helps to prevent constipation too. Of course, if you are using formula milk rather than breastfeeding, it is also vital to take care of yourself and your energy levels, with regular balanced meals and nutritious snacks and drinks.

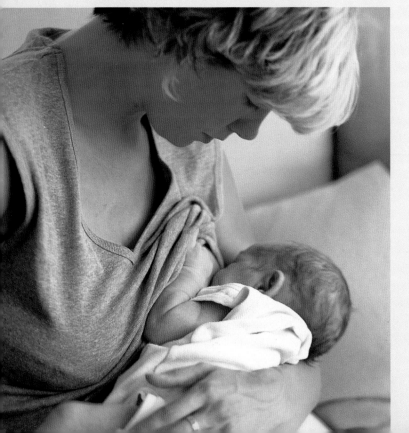

EATING FOR ENERGY

If it seems difficult to find the time to eat properly when you're looking after a young baby, it really helps to:

- ❍ Eat regularly—plan ahead and get help with food shopping and preparation when you can.
- ❍ Eat regular small meals and nutritious snacks and drinks.
- ❍ Keep meals simple so they don't take too long to prepare.
- ❍ Top up energy levels with a smoothie, granola bars, fruit and nuts, or a mug of hearty soup.

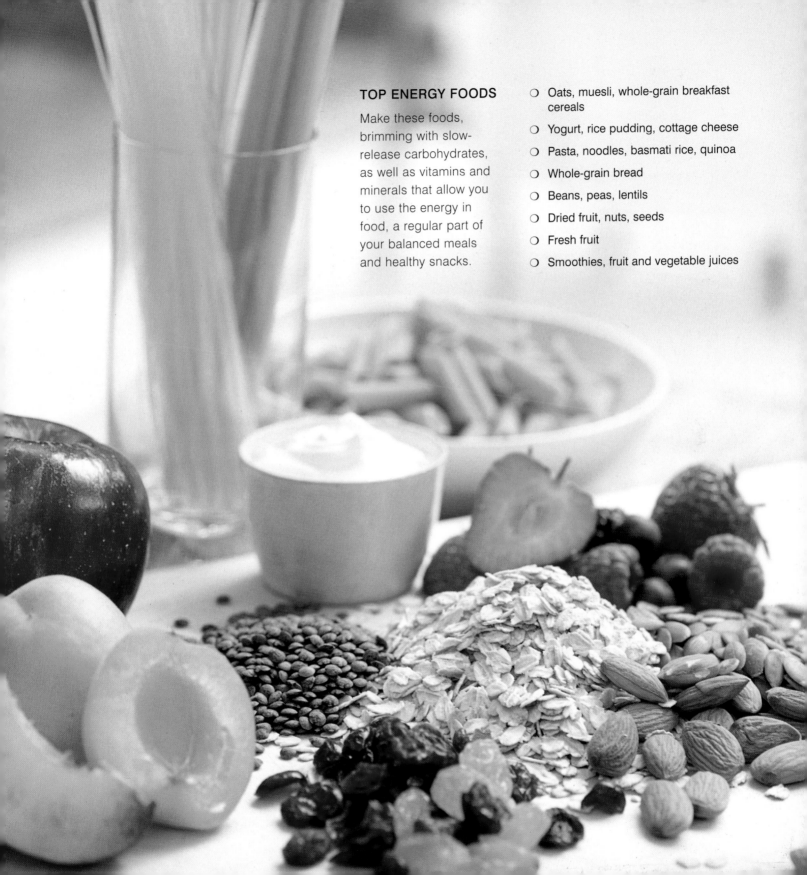

TOP ENERGY FOODS

Make these foods, brimming with slow-release carbohydrates, as well as vitamins and minerals that allow you to use the energy in food, a regular part of your balanced meals and healthy snacks.

- ○ Oats, muesli, whole-grain breakfast cereals
- ○ Yogurt, rice pudding, cottage cheese
- ○ Pasta, noodles, basmati rice, quinoa
- ○ Whole-grain bread
- ○ Beans, peas, lentils
- ○ Dried fruit, nuts, seeds
- ○ Fresh fruit
- ○ Smoothies, fruit and vegetable juices

WHAT TO LIMIT OR AVOID

Your immune system will be functioning effectively again, and as your baby is no longer in direct contact with your blood supply, you can now eat most of the "risky" foods you avoided during pregnancy. But still follow these guidelines while breastfeeding:

❍ Eat no more than two portions of oily fish a week. This advice is for all women who might have a baby one day. Adults are advised to eat no more than one portion of shark, swordfish, or tilefish, and king mackerel a week (*see* page 29).

❍ Keep a limit on drinks containing caffeine (*see* page 29). It passes into breast milk and large amounts can make your baby restless and interfere with their sleep.

❍ You may wish to avoid peanuts if you or the baby's father, brothers, or sisters have an allergic condition such as hay fever, asthma, or eczema.

❍ Alcohol passes into breast milk and can upset your baby. Try to avoid it.

❍ If you have to take any medications, check with your doctor or pharmacist that it is safe while breastfeeding.

WHAT IF A FOOD I EAT AFFECTS MY BABY?

American research has found that a child's future taste preferences can start being shaped by tastes passed on in the womb or during breastfeeding. Therefore, the more varied the mother's diet, the more likely children are to accept a variety of tastes later on. Sometimes babies may seem to react badly to foods their mothers eat. If that happens to you, seek advice from your pediatrician before restricting your diet or cutting out different foods.

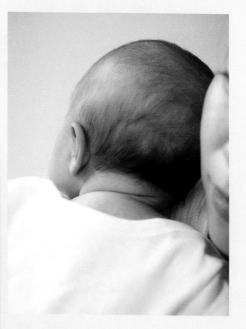

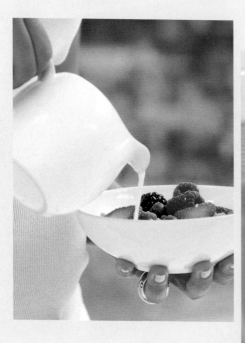

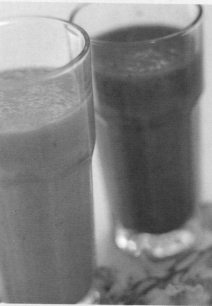

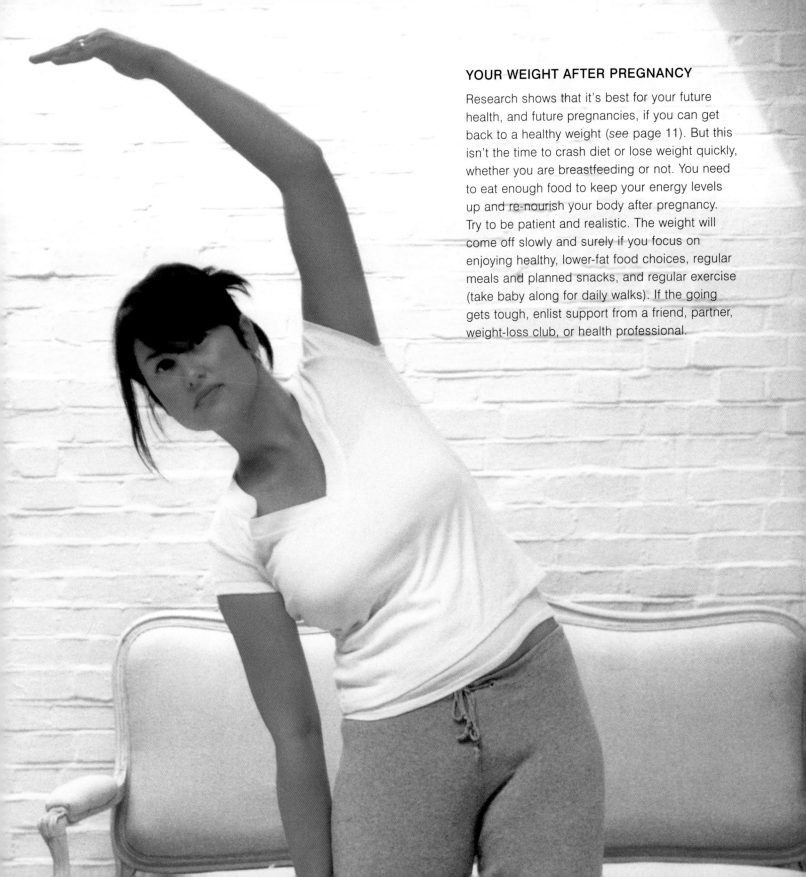

YOUR WEIGHT AFTER PREGNANCY

Research shows that it's best for your future health, and future pregnancies, if you can get back to a healthy weight (see page 11). But this isn't the time to crash diet or lose weight quickly, whether you are breastfeeding or not. You need to eat enough food to keep your energy levels up and re-nourish your body after pregnancy. Try to be patient and realistic. The weight will come off slowly and surely if you focus on enjoying healthy, lower-fat food choices, regular meals and planned snacks, and regular exercise (take baby along for daily walks). If the going gets tough, enlist support from a friend, partner, weight-loss club, or health professional.

Frequently asked questions

Should I exercise while I am pregnant?

Yes, unless there is a medical reason why you shouldn't. Regular gentle to moderate exercise plays an important role in promoting your health and well-being. Women who exercise during pregnancy have healthier weight gains, more rapid weight loss after pregnancy, better general strength and fitness, improved mood and sleep patterns—and a better chance of a straightforward labor. Walking, cycling, and swimming are ideal. This is not the time to take up jerky or very strenuous exercise. If you work out, inform your health club or class instructor that you are pregnant. Make sure you drink plenty of fluids, avoid getting too hot, and stop if you feel unwell. Talk to your doctor or midwife for more individualized information.

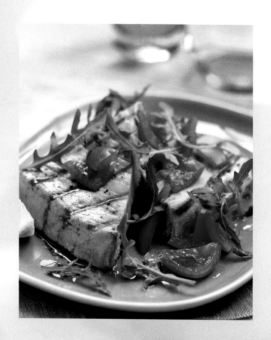

Do I need to avoid peanuts?

Many pregnant women avoid eating peanuts because they are concerned that their baby will develop a peanut allergy. However, in most cases avoiding them is unnecessary. It is generally advised that you may wish to avoid peanuts and peanut products only if you or the baby's father, brothers, or sisters have allergic conditions such as hayfever, asthma, or eczema. Research is ongoing to clarify this issue.

Can certain foods influence the sex of my baby?

Over the centuries there have been numerous anecdotes about how to influence the sex of your baby at conception. When it comes to diet, the approach that has received the most publicity is for women to eat more salty and potassium-rich foods and limit calcium-rich dairy foods for a boy—or eat more dairy foods and limit foods rich in sodium and potassium for a girl. There is no scientific evidence to support this recommendation, and limiting dairy foods or overdoing the salty foods may not be good for your blood pressure or general health. It's best to stick to the conventional approach of "wait and see!"

Can I lose my baby weight in six weeks?

Despite stories of celebrities fitting into their tight jeans again after six weeks, research shows that it can take women without an army of personal trainers and nutritionists an average of 12 months to get back to their pre-pregnancy weight—although much of that is usually lost in the first three months. Remember it took nine months for your weight to increase to support your growing baby, and you need to keep yourself well nourished. Aim to get back to your pre-baby weight gradually with a healthy diet and regular exercise, for your health's sake. Gaining excess weight and not losing it after pregnancy is the most common cause of obesity in women.

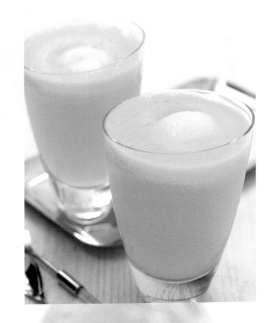

Is it safe to eat Brie and blue-veined cheeses in cooked dishes?

During pregnancy, women are advised not to eat these types of cheese because of the risk of listeria infection. However, thorough cooking should kill any listeria. This means it should be safe to eat food containing soft mold-ripened or blue-veined cheeses, provided it has been properly cooked and is piping hot all the way through.

Should I eat organic food?

Whether or not to eat organic food is really a personal choice. For example, the overall ethos of organic farming, relating to the environment and animal welfare, may be especially important to you. However, the balance of scientific evidence does not support the often-held view that organic food is more nutritious than conventionally grown food. There are also strict controls over the safety and use of pesticides in conventionally produced foods, with both having to meet the same legal food safety requirements.

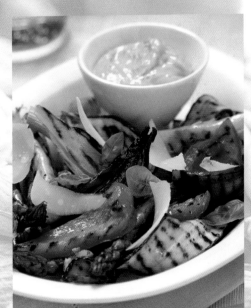

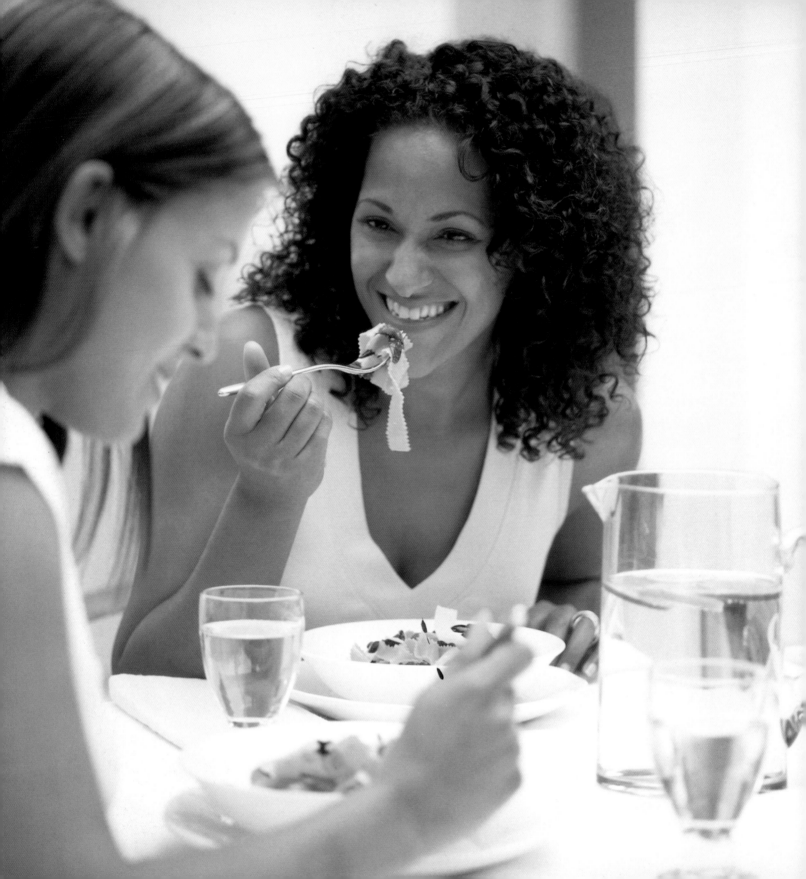

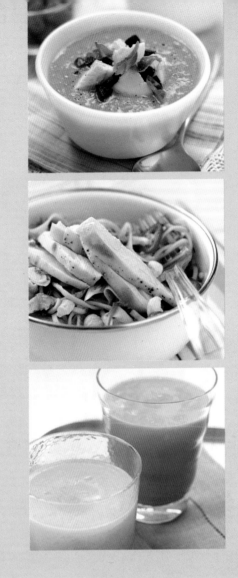

RECIPES

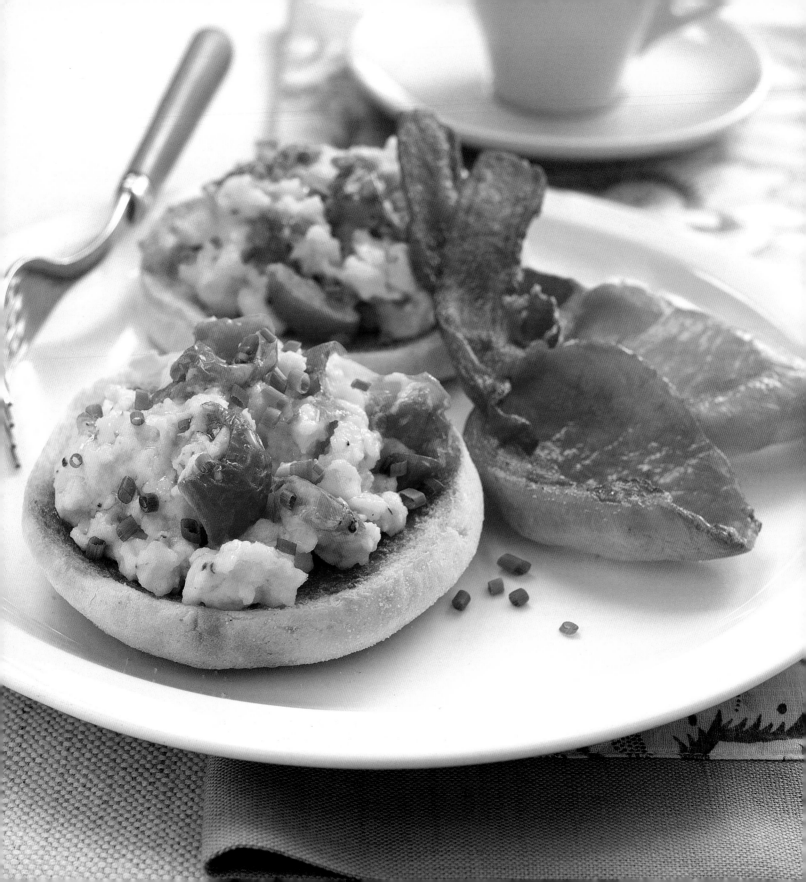

breakfasts and brunches

breakfast bruschetta

Eggs make a nutritious start to the day, providing vital protein, B vitamins, vitamin D, and zinc, but it is important that they are cooked thoroughly while you are pregnant to avoid the possible risk of salmonella.

2 slices lean bacon

2 oz. half-dried tomatoes

2 tablespoons low-fat milk

2 large free-range eggs, lightly beaten

2 teaspoons unsalted butter

1 whole-wheat English muffin, halved horizontally

1 tablespoon snipped fresh chives (optional)

sea salt and freshly ground black pepper

SERVES 1

Preheat the broiler to medium and line the broiler pan with foil. Cook the bacon until crisp. Keep warm.

Meanwhile, if using half-dried tomatoes in oil, rinse them under cold running water, then pat dry using paper towels. Snip the tomatoes into bite-size pieces.

Beat the milk into the eggs and season to taste, then toast the muffin halves.

Heat the butter in a small nonstick saucepan and add the half-dried tomatoes and egg mixture. Using a wooden spoon, stir the egg mixture constantly but gently to ensure it doesn't stick to the pan. Cook for about 2 minutes, or until the eggs are scrambled and cooked through.

Spoon the eggs on top of each muffin half and sprinkle with the chives, if using. Serve with the bacon.

VARIATION
In place of the half-dried tomatoes, use 1–2 vine-ripened tomatoes (depending on size), seeded and roughly chopped, or some red bell pepper, seeded and diced.

maple almond crisp

It is important to include a good range of essential fatty acids in our diet. The variety of nuts and seeds in this recipe provides a nourishing mix of both omega-3 and omega-6 fatty acids. The oats and dried fruit help to make it a slow energy release breakfast or snack.

½ cup whole blanched almonds

1½ cups old-fashioned rolled oats

⅓ cup sesame seeds

⅓ cup sunflower seeds, hulled

¼ cup pumpkin seeds

3 tablespoons sunflower oil

7 tablespoons pure maple syrup or clear honey (or a mixture of both)

⅓ cup walnut pieces

½ cup unsulfured dried apricots, roughly chopped

TO SERVE

thick, low-fat yogurt
or low-fat milk

fresh fruit, such as sliced strawberries, apple or banana, or whole blueberries and raspberries

MAKES ABOUT 10 PORTIONS

2 baking sheets with sides, greased

Preheat the oven to 275°F.

Put the almonds, oats, and seeds in a large bowl.

Heat the oil and maple syrup in a saucepan over medium heat, stirring until melted and mixed together. Add the almonds, oats, and seeds to the pan, then mix well until they are thoroughly coated in the maple syrup mixture.

Spoon onto the 2 baking sheets in an even layer and bake in the preheated oven for 15 minutes. Remove from the oven and sprinkle over the walnuts. Stir carefully until combined.

Return the baking sheets to the oven and cook for another 10 minutes until golden and slightly crisp. (The mixture will become crisper as it cools.)

Transfer the cereal to a bowl and add the chopped apricots. Mix well and let cool. Transfer to an airtight container.

To serve, pour the cereal into a bowl and spoon over the yogurt or pour over milk. Top with fresh fruit of your choice.

VARIATION

Any of your favorite nuts, seeds, grains, or dried fruit can be used in this recipe.

Nuts and seeds

Nuts and seeds contain a wide range of nutrients vital for a healthy pregnancy. They make a great snack, ingredient, or topping for salads, yogurt, or cereal. For optimal benefits, enjoy a mix of nuts and seeds. As well as being nutritious, all have unique benefits. Pumpkin seeds and walnuts in this recipe provide omega-3 fats (*see page 17*), the sunflower seeds burst with vitamin E and selenium, and the sesame seeds and almonds provide calcium.

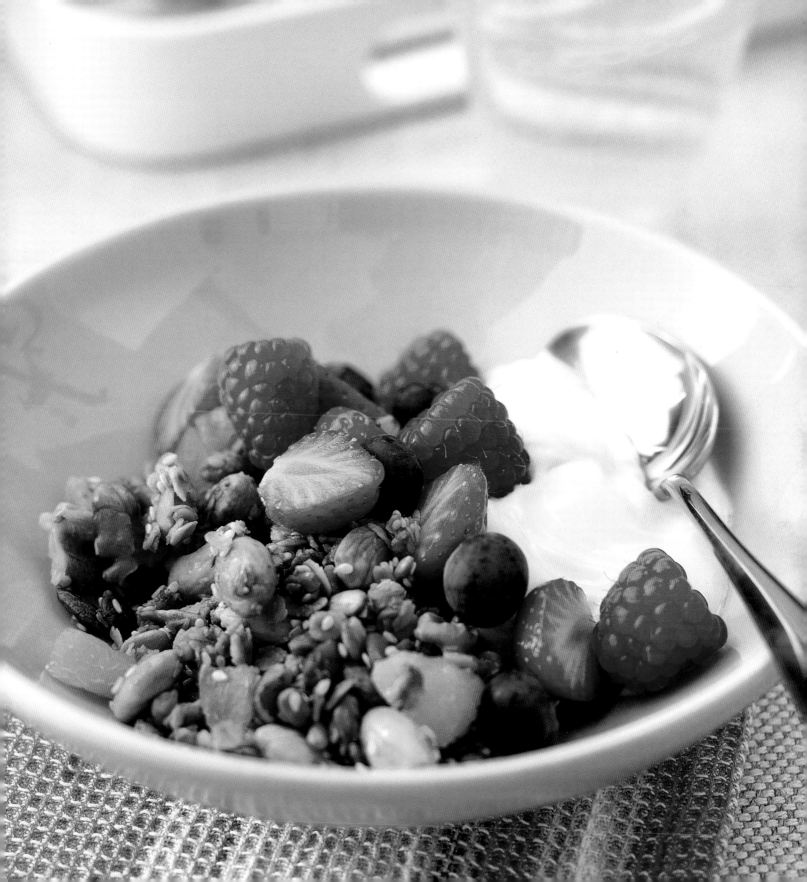

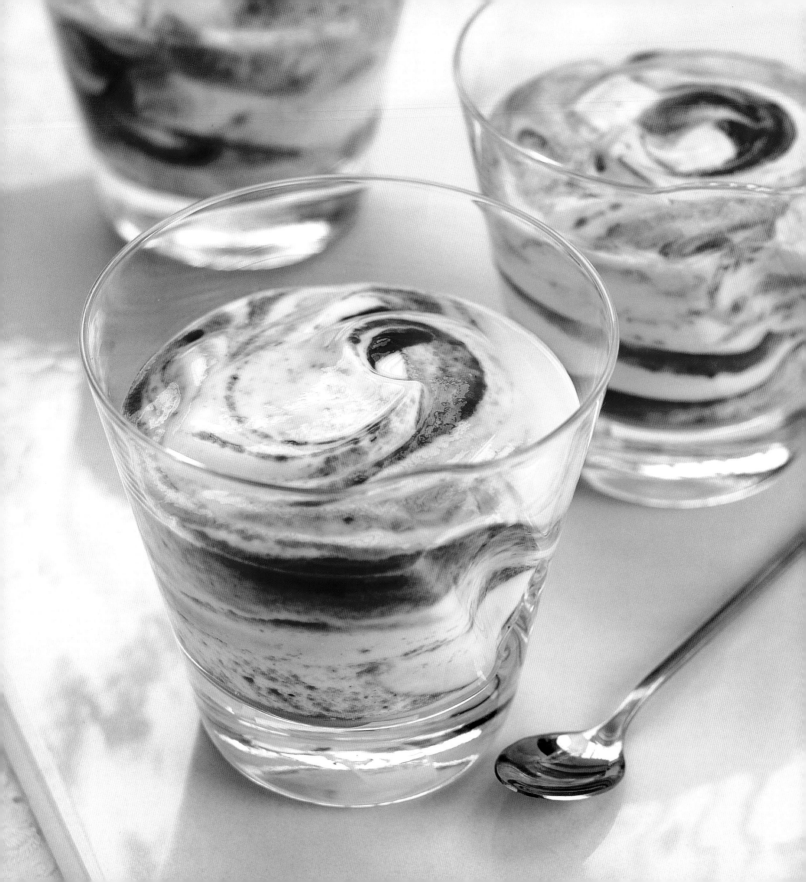

yogurt and summer fruit swirl

If fresh fruit is not in season, use frozen fruit instead, which still counts toward the recommended "five-a-day" (*see* page 62). Any leftover fruit purée can be stored for two days in an airtight container in the fridge or frozen.

1 cup (5 oz.) frozen mixed red berries

3 ripe purple plums, halved, pitted, and chopped

1 tablespoon confectioners' sugar, or to taste

thick, plain low-fat yogurt, to serve

SERVES 2

Put the frozen berries in a saucepan with the plums and ½ cup water. Bring up to simmering point, then cover the pan and cook for 5–7 minutes until they soften and begin to break down.

Transfer the fruit and any juice to a blender or food processor and process until smooth, then press through a strainer to remove any seeds. Stir in the confectioners' sugar and taste the fruit purée for sweetness; add more confectioners' sugar if it is too tart.

Spoon 3–4 tablespoons of yogurt into a glass or bowl. Add a few spoonfuls of the fruit purée and swirl it into the yogurt using a spoon handle to give a marbled effect.

VARIATION: DRIED APRICOT PURÉE
Dried fruit purées can be adapted to suit your taste, and are a good source of iron. Put ⅔ cup unsulfured dried apricots, ⅔ cup apple juice, and ⅔ cup water in a pan. Bring to a boil, cover, then reduce the heat and simmer for 20 minutes. Purée the apricots and liquid in a blender or food processor until smooth, then let cool.

porridge with cinnamon plums

Full of valuable fiber, vitamins, and minerals, porridge is wonderfully comforting and sustaining, while the stewed plums add natural sweetness along with antioxidants.

¾ cup old-fashioned rolled oats

1⅔ cups low-fat milk

a pinch of salt

a drizzle of pure maple syrup and some chopped pistachio nuts, to serve

CINNAMON PLUMS

4 slightly firm red plums, quartered

½ cup fresh apple or orange juice (not from concentrate)

1 cinnamon stick

SERVES 2

Put the oats in a saucepan with the milk, salt, and 1¼ cups water. Bring to a boil, then reduce the heat and simmer, half-covered, for 4–5 minutes, stirring frequently.

For the cinnamon plums, put the plums, apple juice, and cinnamon in a small saucepan and cook, covered, for 4–5 minutes over medium-low heat until the plums are tender and the juice reduced and thickened.

To serve, divide the porridge between 2 bowls, then spoon over the plums and a little of the sauce, discarding the cinnamon. Drizzle with maple syrup and a sprinkling of pistachio nuts.

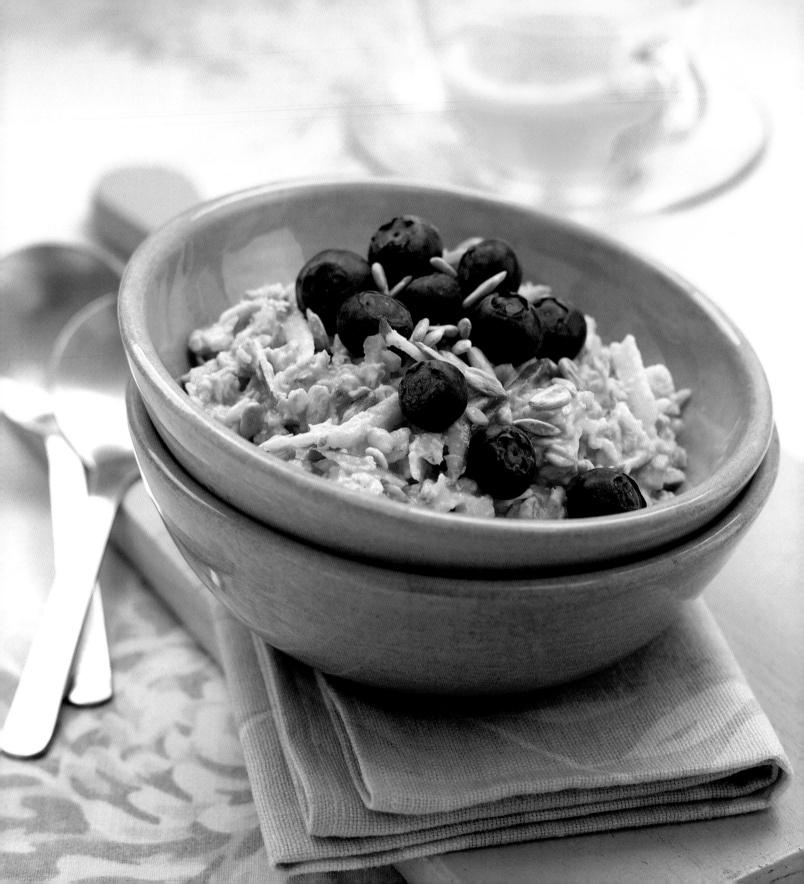

blueberry and apple bircher muesli

Blueberries are bursting with beneficial antioxidants, and the oats, apples, and seeds provide fiber and slow release energy to keep you going through the morning.

2 cups old-fashioned rolled oats

1 cup fresh apple juice (not from concentrate)

⅓ cup low-fat milk

½ cup thick, plain low-fat yogurt

1 apple, cored and grated

blueberries and toasted sunflower seeds, to serve

SERVES 2–3

Put the oats in a mixing bowl and pour the apple juice over. Cover the bowl with plastic wrap and leave in the fridge overnight.

Just before serving, stir in the milk, yogurt, and grated apple. Spoon into bowls and top with blueberries and toasted sunflower seeds.

Apples

Women who ate more than four apples a week during pregnancy halved the risk of their child being diagnosed with asthma compared to mothers-to-be who ate the least apples, according to a study from the University of Aberdeen, Scotland. Other studies have also linked regular apple eating with better lung health, possibly because of the beneficial mix of antioxidants they contain.

winter fruit compote

Dried fruit is not only brimming with fiber, but also provides energy-giving natural sugars and iron (especially figs and apricots). Brazil nuts contain more selenium (good for the immune system and thyroid function) than any other food.

1½ cups mixed dried fruit, such as figs, prunes, apricots, pears, and apple

1 cup fresh orange juice (not from concentrate)

1 teaspoon apple pie spice

low-fat Greek yogurt or cottage cheese and chopped Brazil nuts, to serve

SERVES 2–3

Put the dried fruit in a bowl and cover with water. Set aside to soak for 6 hours or overnight.

Drain the fruit and put it in a saucepan with the orange juice and apple pie spice. Bring to a boil, then reduce the heat, half-cover, and simmer for 20 minutes until the fruit becomes plump and tender and the liquid has reduced and become syrupy.

Serve the compote warm or cold, topped with a dollop of Greek yogurt and a sprinkling of chopped Brazil nuts.

cottage cheese pancakes
with sweet chili mushrooms

Not only is cottage cheese low in fat, it adds extra protein to these pancakes as well as providing valuable calcium for teeth and bones. The batter makes about 15 pancakes—obviously too many for two people, but the remainder can be chilled or frozen for future use.

Put the flour, eggs, milk, cottage cheese, and salt in a food processor and process to a smooth batter. Set the batter aside for 30 minutes to rest.

Lightly oil a large nonstick skillet and ladle the batter into the skillet to form a round pancake—you will probably be able to cook 3 pancakes at a time. Cook the pancakes for 1½–2 minutes per side until golden.

Keep the pancakes you've already made warm while you make the rest. When all the batter is used, wipe the skillet clean, then add 1 tablespoon oil. Fry the mushrooms for about 5 minutes until tender, then remove from the heat and stir in the sweet chili sauce and 1 tablespoon water.

To serve, put 3 pancakes on each plate and top with the mushrooms. Spoon over any sauce left in the pan.

VARIATION: COTTAGE CHEESE AND CORN PANCAKES
Stir ¾ cup corn kernels (frozen or canned) into the batter mixture after it has rested. The corn pancakes are delicious with bacon and a drizzle of maple syrup.

1⅓ cups self-rising flour

2 large free-range eggs

1¼ cups low-fat milk

½ cup cottage cheese

a large pinch of sea salt

sunflower or canola oil, for frying

SWEET CHILI MUSHROOMS

2 large flat mushrooms, sliced

2–3 tablespoons sweet chili sauce

SERVES 2

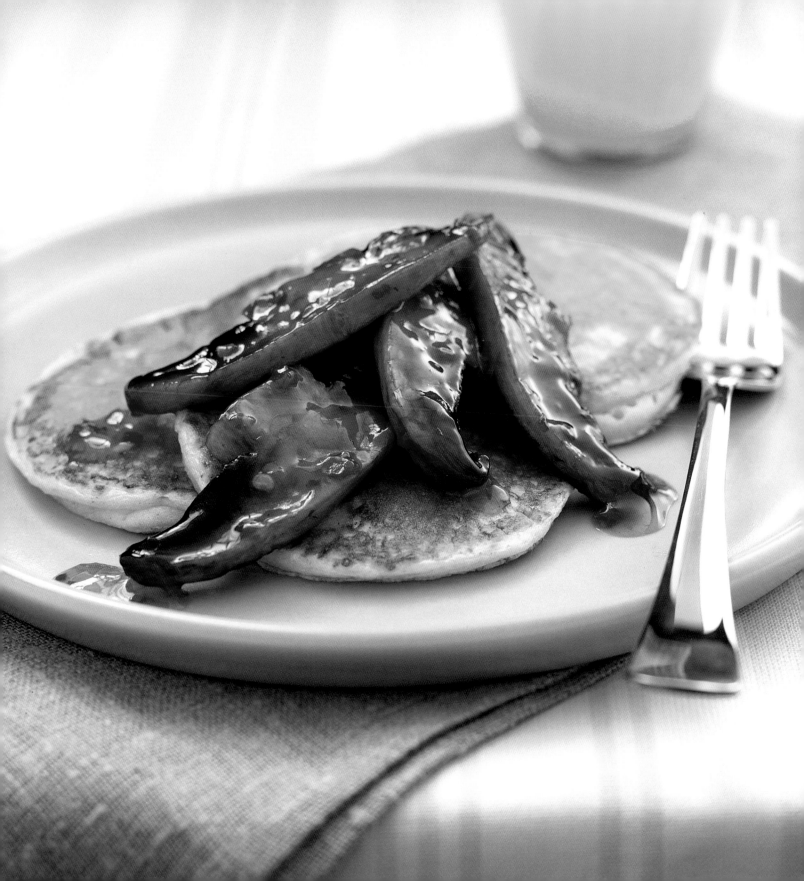

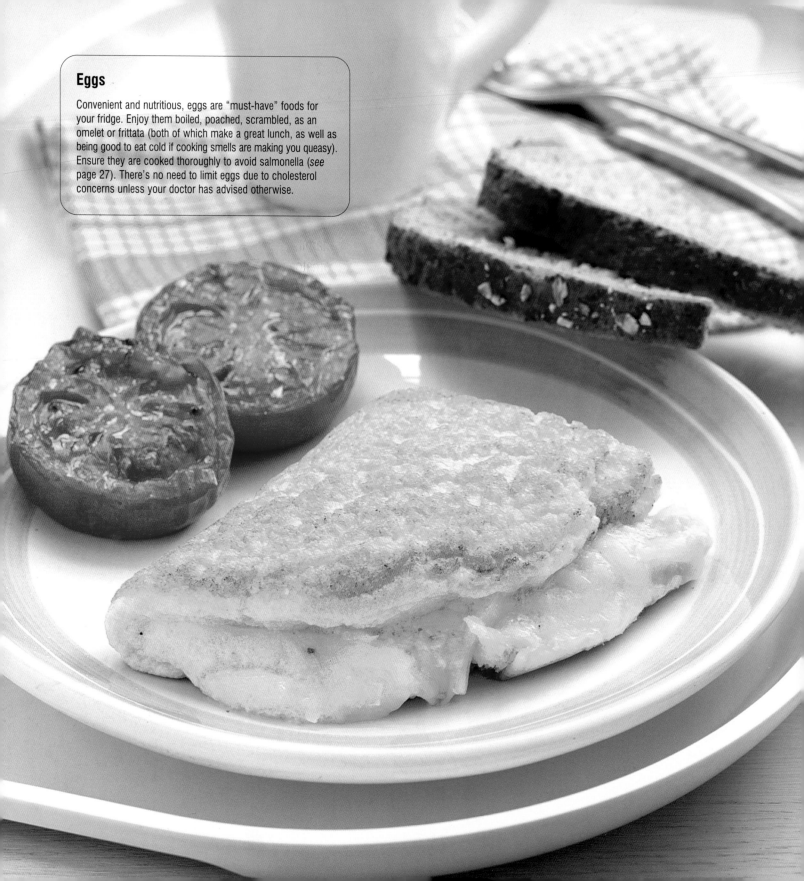

Eggs

Convenient and nutritious, eggs are "must-have" foods for your fridge. Enjoy them boiled, poached, scrambled, as an omelet or frittata (both of which make a great lunch, as well as being good to eat cold if cooking smells are making you queasy). Ensure they are cooked thoroughly to avoid salmonella (*see* page 27). There's no need to limit eggs due to cholesterol concerns unless your doctor has advised otherwise.

soufflé cheese omelet

A great brunch or light lunch; the whisked egg whites give this omelet a light, fluffy texture. Folic acid and vitamin B_{12} are both found in eggs, and they work together to help a baby's spinal cord develop normally in the early stages of pregnancy. Serve with whole-grain bread.

2 large free-range eggs, separated

sea salt and freshly ground black pepper

1 vine-ripened tomato, halved horizontally

a pat of butter

½ cup grated sharp cheddar

SERVES 1–2

Preheat the broiler to medium. Line the broiler pan with foil.

Meanwhile, beat the egg whites in a large, clean bowl until they form stiff peaks. Season the egg yolks and beat them in a separate bowl until even in color and texture. Carefully fold the egg whites into the egg yolks using a metal spoon.

Put the tomato under the broiler and cook for 6–8 minutes, turning once. After the tomato has been cooking for 4 minutes, heat the butter in a medium nonstick skillet. When the butter has melted, swirl it around the skillet to cover the base.

Tip the egg mixture into the skillet and flatten gently with a spatula until it covers the base of the skillet. Cook over medium heat for 2 minutes, then sprinkle the cheese over the center of the omelet. Cook for another minute, or until the base is light golden.

Carefully fold the omelet in half to encase the cheese. When the egg is set, slide onto a plate. The omelet is large and will satisfy 1 hungry person, or cut in half will feed 2 people. Serve with the broiled tomato.

bubble and squeak patties

A great way of using up leftover mashed potatoes, these patties contain two of nature's overlooked wonder foods—cabbage and potatoes—which both supply vitamin C and folic acid. Serve the patties with broiled tomatoes and chicken or vegetarian sausages. They're also good cold as a snack.

1 cup shredded Savoy cabbage

1½ cups mashed potatoes

¼ cup grated sharp cheddar

1½ teaspoons Dijon mustard

1 small free-range egg, lightly beaten

flour, for dusting

2 tablespoons sunflower or canola oil

sea salt and freshly ground black pepper

MAKES 6

Steam the cabbage for 2–3 minutes until just tender. Let cool, then squeeze out any excess water using your hands.

Finely chop the cabbage, then put it in a bowl with the mashed potatoes, cheese, and Dijon mustard. Season to taste and mix until combined, then stir in the egg.

Divide the mixture into 6. Using floured hands, form each portion into a patty shape. Lightly dust each patty with flour.

Pour the oil into a large nonstick skillet and heat. Cook 3 patties at a time for 3–4 minutes each side until golden, adding a little more oil if necessary. Keep the cakes that you've cooked warm while you cook the rest. Drain the patties on paper towels to remove any excess oil before serving.

melon and ginger wake-up

Melon and ginger are natural partners, and orange-fleshed melons are richer in vitamin C and beta-carotene than other varieties. Ginger is known for its anti-nausea benefits and people often find melon easier to manage than other fruits if they feel a bit queasy.

Put the ginger and melon through a juicer, stir, and pour the juice into 2 glasses.

VARIATION
In place of the melon, substitute 1 small pineapple, halved, skin removed, cored, and cut into wedges. Put through a juicer with the ginger and stir before serving.

1 inch fresh ginger

1 cantaloupe, cut into thin wedges, seeded and skin removed

SERVES 2

date and vanilla smoothie

This smoothie tastes so rich and indulgent, it's hard to believe it's good for you. A nourishing and energy-boosting blend of protein and slow-release carbohydrate, it makes an excellent start to the day.

Put the dates and 1¼ cups water in a saucepan. Bring to a boil, then reduce the heat and simmer, covered, for 10 minutes until the dates are soft. Let cool.

Put the dates and any remaining water, yogurt, vanilla, and milk in a blender. Blend until smooth and creamy. Pour into 2 glasses.

5 oz. pitted dates, roughly chopped

½ cup thick, plain low-fat yogurt

1 teaspoon pure vanilla extract

1¼ cups low-fat milk

SERVES 2

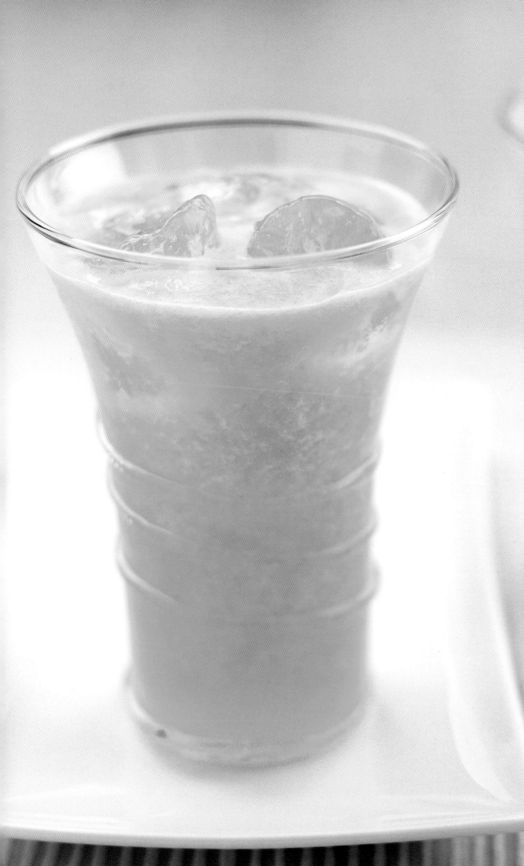

peach and orange nectar

You can select nectarines or peaches for this recipe, both of which add richness to the juice as well as providing a vitamin C boost. It may also be easier to manage than orange juice if you have heartburn.

5 ripe peaches or nectarines, halved, pitted, and quartered

3 oranges, halved horizontally

ice, to serve (optional)

SERVES 2

Put the peaches through a juicer.

Use a citrus press or hand-held juicer to squeeze the juice from the oranges. Stir together the peach and orange juices, then pour into two glasses. Add ice, if liked.

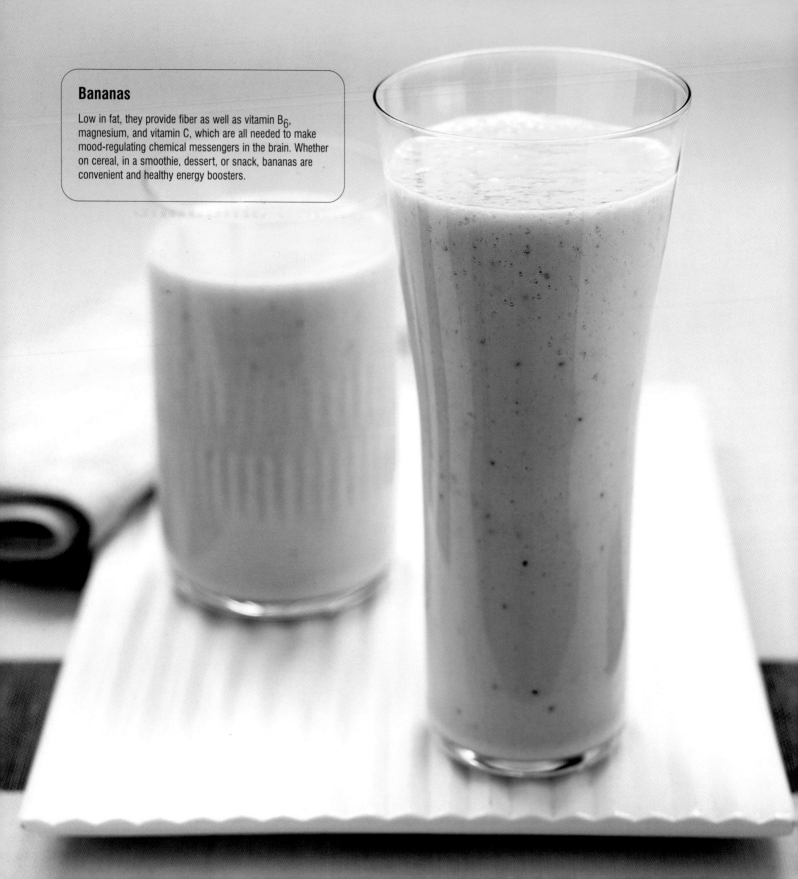

Bananas

Low in fat, they provide fiber as well as vitamin B_6, magnesium, and vitamin C, which are all needed to make mood-regulating chemical messengers in the brain. Whether on cereal, in a smoothie, dessert, or snack, bananas are convenient and healthy energy boosters.

almond and banana shake

Protein-rich milk and almonds combine to provide beneficial amounts of the antioxidant vitamin E, B vitamins, and healthy oils and minerals, including bone-building calcium. The almonds also add a wonderful creaminess.

½ cup whole blanched almonds

1⅔ cups low-fat milk

2 ripe bananas, thickly sliced

1 teaspoon pure vanilla extract

freshly grated nutmeg, to serve

SERVES 2

Put the almonds in a food processor or blender and process until finely ground.

Add the milk, bananas, and vanilla, then blend until smooth and creamy. Pour into 2 glasses and sprinkle a little nutmeg over the top.

strawberry and banana smoothie

Satisfying and filling, this smoothie is full of vital nutrients and energy to kick-start your day. The milk and yogurt provide calcium, protein, and B vitamins, while the fruit serves up vitamin C and magnesium, both essential for healthy bones and teeth.

2 bananas

2 cups strawberries, hulled

½ teaspoon pure vanilla extract (optional)

⅔ cup thick, plain low-fat yogurt

1½ cups low-fat milk

SERVES 2

Slice the bananas and put them in a blender with the strawberries, vanilla, if using, yogurt, and milk.

Blend until the mixture is thick, smooth, and creamy. Pour the smoothie into 2 glasses.

breakfast juice

If you can't face solid food first thing, this nutritious and soothing drink combines fruit and vegetables to get you going in the morning. However, make sure you follow it with a snack. For maximum goodness, it's important to drink the juice soon after making it, since vitamins start to diminish once fruit and vegetables are cut.

4 apples, stalks removed

2 large carrots, scrubbed

1 inch fresh ginger

squeeze of fresh lemon juice

SERVES 2

Cut the apples into quarters and halve the carrots. Put the apples, carrots, and ginger through a juicer.

Pour the juice into 2 glasses and stir in a squeeze of lemon juice.

pineapple and citrus juice

This vibrant juice is a real wake-up drink and is bursting with vitamin C. Making it part of breakfast will boost iron absorption from your cereal, toast, or baked beans. For a longer drink, dilute with sparkling or still mineral water.

1 small pineapple, halved lengthwise, peeled, cored, and cut into long wedges

2 oranges, halved horizontally

1 red grapefruit, halved horizontally

SERVES 2

Put the pineapple through a juicer.

Use a citrus press or hand-held juicer to squeeze the juice from the oranges and grapefruit.

Mix together the pineapple and citrus juices in a jug and pour into 2 glasses.

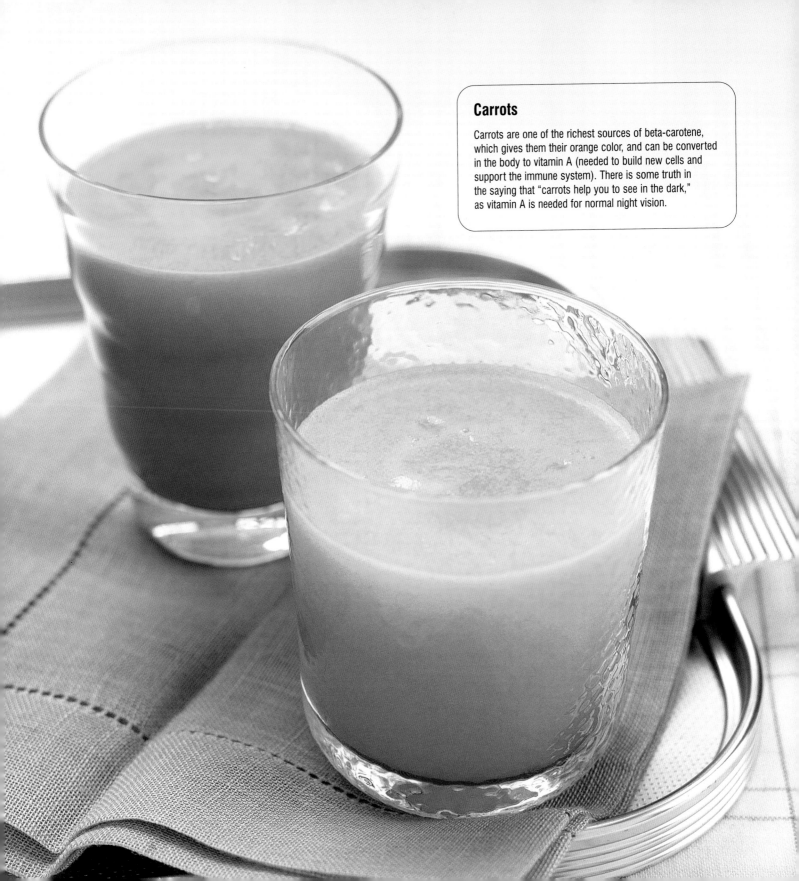

Carrots

Carrots are one of the richest sources of beta-carotene, which gives them their orange color, and can be converted in the body to vitamin A (needed to build new cells and support the immune system). There is some truth in the saying that "carrots help you to see in the dark," as vitamin A is needed for normal night vision.

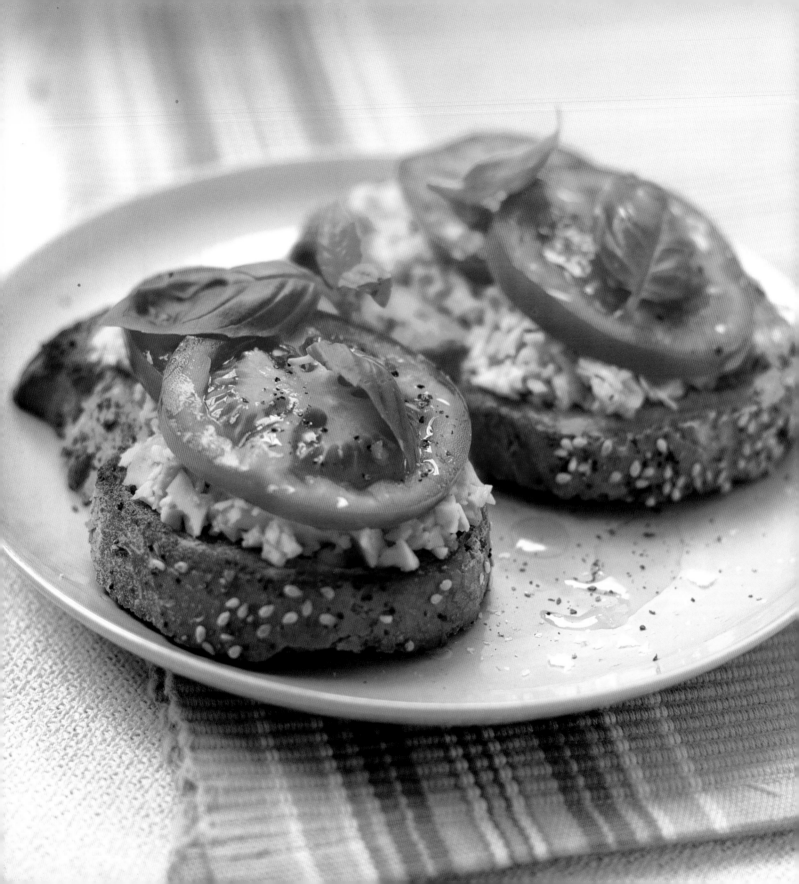

avocado and tomato toast

The success of this simple and nutritious snack relies on the quality of the ingredients: make sure the tomatoes have plenty of flavor and the avocado is ripe to perfection. This is best eaten soon after making, and can also be served as a light lunch with a green salad.

2 thick slices of walnut or whole-grain bread

1 small avocado, halved and pitted

½ teaspoon balsamic vinegar or lemon juice

1 vine-ripened tomato, sliced

extra virgin olive oil, for drizzling

4 large fresh basil leaves

sea salt and freshly ground black pepper

SERVES 2 OR 1 AS
A LIGHT LUNCH

Toast the walnut bread on both sides.

Scoop the avocado flesh out of its skin with a spoon, then mash with the balsamic vinegar. Spoon the avocado onto the toast—there's no need for any butter.

Top the avocado with the slices of tomato and drizzle with a little extra virgin olive oil. Season with salt and freshly ground black pepper, then scatter with the basil leaves.

Whole-grain bread

Opt for whole-grain bread whenever you can. It is great for bowel-regulating fiber, as well as B vitamins and minerals. Grainy types provide slow-release energy. Studies also suggest that eating three or more servings of whole-grain foods daily is linked to a reduced risk of type 2 diabetes, obesity, and coronary heart disease.

mozzarella and tuna quesadilla

Irresistible and satisfying, this golden tortilla parcel is filled with melted protein-rich mozzarella and tuna. Diced sweet bell pepper, chopped scallions, or herbs, such as chives can also be added, if liked.

olive oil, for brushing

2 large whole-wheat or soft tortillas

3½ oz. canned tuna in spring water, drained and mashed with a fork

6 slices of mozzarella, about 2½ oz. total weight

10 fresh basil leaves

freshly ground black pepper

SERVES 2–4

Lightly brush a large nonstick skillet with oil. Put one tortilla into the skillet so it fits snugly. Spoon the tuna over the tortilla, leaving a 1-inch gap around the edge. Top the tuna with the mozzarella and basil, then season with pepper to taste.

Put the second tortilla on top of the filling, pressing it down around the edges. Put the skillet over medium-low heat and cook the quesadilla for 3 minutes until the tortilla is golden and beginning to crisp.

To cook the other side of the quesadilla, put a large plate on top of the skillet and carefully flip it over to release the quesadilla onto the plate, then slide it back into the skillet. Cook the tortilla for another 3 minutes until golden and the mozzarella is melted.

Slide the quesadilla onto a serving plate, let it cool slightly, then cut into 6 wedges.

Different cheeses

Cheese provides protein and bone-building calcium, and suitable types (see page 27) are great to include throughout pregnancy. Typically, weight for weight, hard cheeses, such as cheddar and Parmesan, provide more calcium, but are higher in fat than soft cheeses, such as cottage or ricotta. Most medium-fat cheeses, such as mozzarella and halloumi, provide a medium amount of calcium, while Gouda and Edam also have a medium fat content, but are as rich in calcium as cheddar. To optimize nutrition, vary your cheeses, and keep in check portion sizes (see page 13).

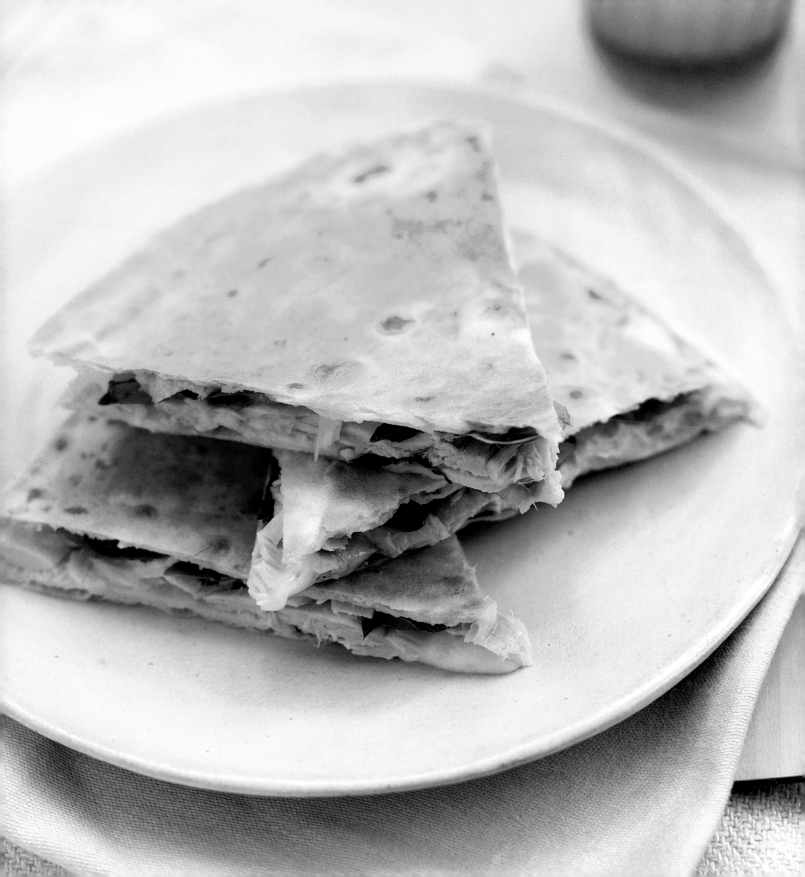

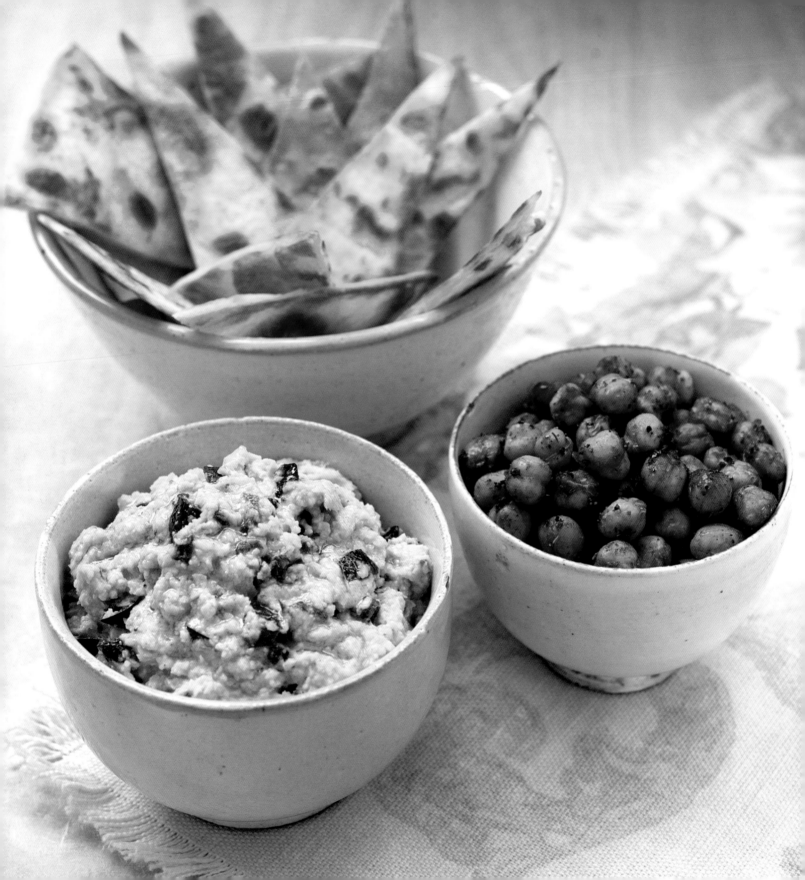

olive hummus
with tortilla dippers

This chickpea dip makes a welcome change to storebought versions.

14-oz. can chickpeas
(about 8 oz. drained weight)

freshly squeezed juice of 1 lemon

2 garlic cloves, crushed

2 tablespoons tahini (sesame seed) paste

3 tablespoons extra virgin olive oil

2 oz. pitted black olives, finely chopped

1 soft tortilla, cut into wedges

sea salt and freshly ground black pepper

MAKES ABOUT 10 SERVINGS

Drain and rinse the chickpeas, then put them in a food processor with the lemon juice, garlic, tahini paste, olive oil, and 2 tablespoons water. Process until puréed, but still a little chunky—you will have to stir the hummus occasionally during blending to keep the mixture moving. Add an extra tablespoon water, if necessary, and season well with salt and pepper.

Spoon the hummus into an airtight container and stir in the olives. Put the tortilla wedges into a dry skillet and cook for a few minutes, turning once, until crisp. Serve with the hummus.

roasted Cajun chickpeas

When roasted in a Cajun-spiced oil, chickpeas are transformed into crunchy little nuggets and make a nutritious nibble.

14-oz. can chickpeas
(about 240 g
drained weight)

1 tablespoon olive oil

½ teaspoon sea salt

1–2 teaspoons
Cajun spice mix

SERVES 4

Preheat the oven to 325°F. Drain and rinse the chickpeas. Line a plate with paper towels and pour the chickpeas on top. Lay another sheet of paper towels on top and pat dry.

Tip the chickpeas into a small mixing bowl and add the oil, salt, and Cajun spice mix. Stir until the chickpeas are coated in the spicy oil mixture.

Spread the chickpeas over a baking sheet with sides in an even layer and roast for 1 hour, or until crisp. Remove from the oven and let cool. Store for up to 3 days in an airtight container.

soy-toasted nuts and seeds

Nuts are great for protein, iron, vitamin E, selenium, and fiber. While they tend to be high in fat, it is mostly the healthy unsaturated type. Seeds are nutritious too, with pumpkin seeds providing both omega-3 and omega-6 fatty acids.

6½ oz. mixed unsalted nuts and seeds, such as walnuts, Brazil nuts, almonds, cashews, hazelnuts, sunflower seeds, and pumpkin seeds

1 tablespoon soy sauce

MAKES 6½ OZ. (A SMALL HANDFUL IS ABOUT 1 OZ.; A GOOD SNACK SIZE)

Preheat the oven to 325°F.

Spread out your chosen selection of nuts on a baking sheet with sides and roast for about 6 minutes.

Add the seeds and turn until combined. Roast for another 2–4 minutes until they smell toasted and are light golden. Keep an eye on them, as they burn easily.

Remove the nuts and seeds from the oven and transfer them to a bowl. Let cool slightly, then drizzle the soy sauce over the top, and turn the nuts and seeds with a spoon until they are coated.

fruit and nut mix

You can find small bags of trail mix in most supermarkets, but more often than not they contain extra sugar or oil. There is also the possibility that you won't like the ready-made combination of fruit and nuts. Feel free to choose your own favorite combinations, using the recipe below as a guide.

3 tablespoons sunflower seeds

3 tablespoons pumpkin seeds

2 oz. dried mango pieces or figs

2 oz. unsulfured dried apricots

1 oz. walnuts or hazelnuts

1 oz. Brazil nuts or cashews

2 tablespoons hemp seeds
or flaxseed

MAKES ABOUT 4–5 PORTIONS

Put the sunflower and pumpkin seeds in a dry skillet and cook over medium-low heat, tossing the seeds occasionally, until they are lightly toasted—keep an eye on them, as they can easily burn. Let cool.

Roughly chop the mango pieces and quarter the apricots. Halve the walnuts and Brazil nuts.

Put the toasted seeds, hemp seeds, dried fruit, and nuts in an airtight container and mix well. Store for up to 1 week.

What counts as a fruit or vegetable portion?

Dried fruit can count toward the recommended five portions of fruit and vegetables per day.

A portion could be:

- 1 medium piece of fruit e.g. orange, apple, banana

- 1 small can of fruit in juice, or 3 tablespoons stewed or canned fruit

- 2 small fruits e.g. clementines, plums

- 1 large slice of a large fruit e.g. pineapple, melon

- 1 tablespoon dried fruit

- 5-oz. glass pure juice (count this just once toward your five a day)

- 3 tablespoons vegetables—fresh, frozen, or canned (excluding potatoes)

- 1 cereal bowlful of salad

---

pesto and mozzarella toastie

A variation on classic cheese on toast, but with an Italian twist. Mozzarella is lower in fat than cheddar, but remains a good source of calcium and protein.

1 ciabatta roll, halved horizontally

1–2 teaspoons red pesto

4 thin slices of mozzarella

freshly ground black pepper

SERVES 1

Preheat the broiler to medium. Lightly toast the uncut side of each half of the ciabatta roll.

Turn the ciabatta halves over and spread with the pesto. Top with the mozzarella and return it to the broiler. Cook for about 3 minutes until the mozzarella melts and begins to color.

Season with freshly ground black pepper before serving.

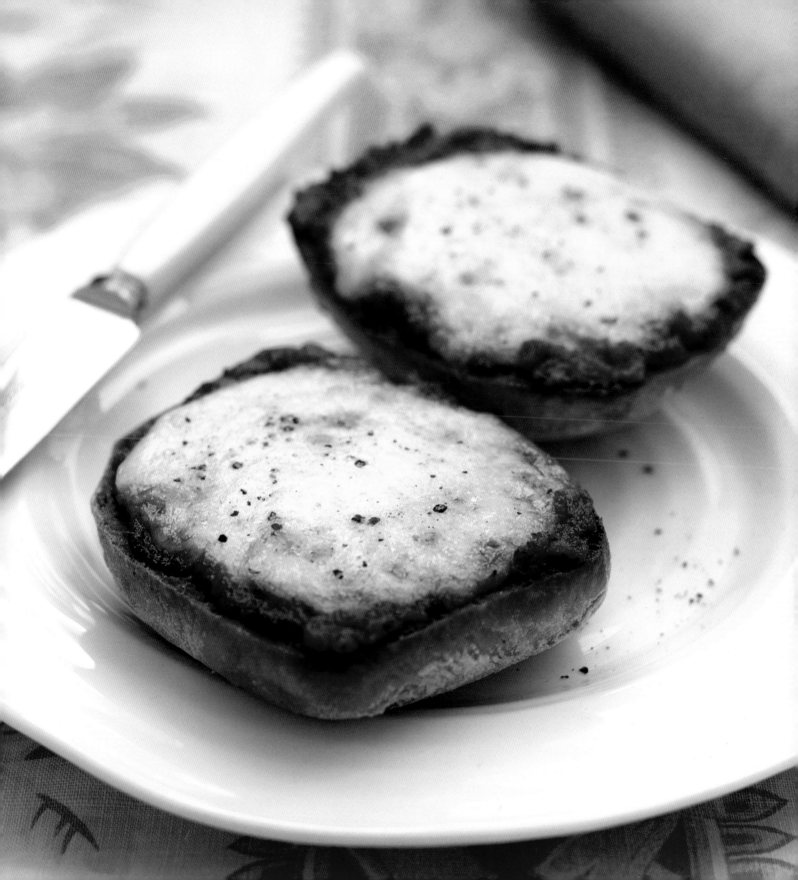

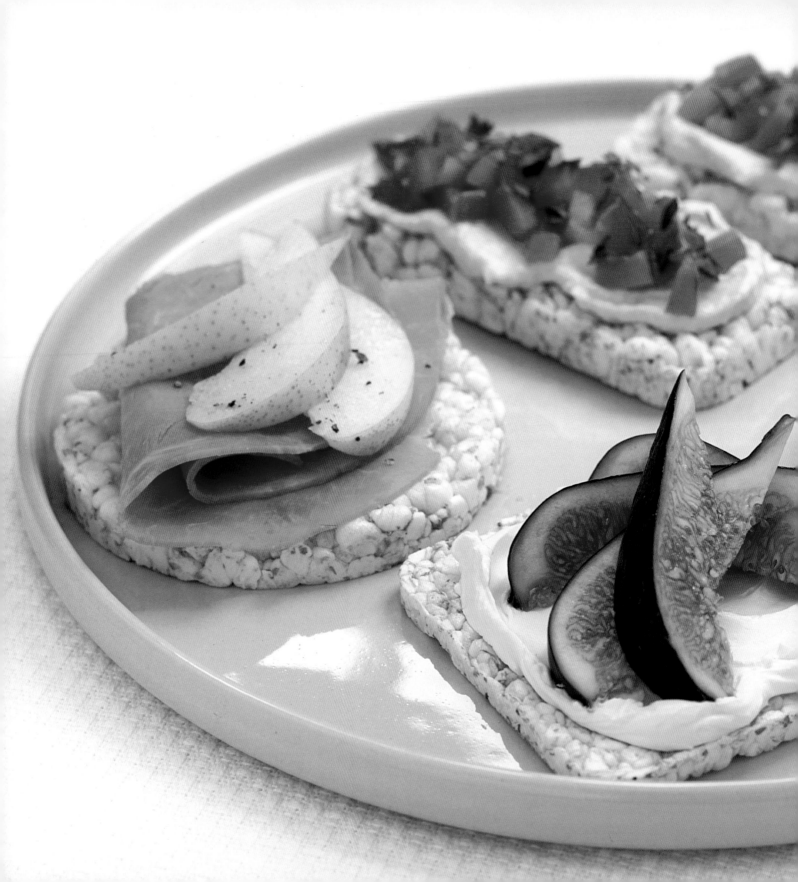

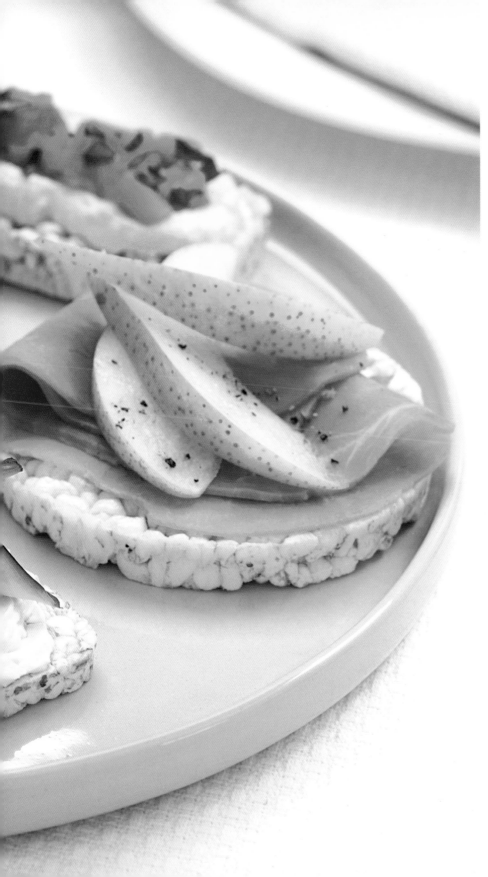

rice cakes with toppings

Rice cakes form an ideal base for a wide range of sweet and savory toppings, and make a pleasant change to bread, toasted or otherwise, or other types of crackers. Try to choose plain, whole-grain rice cakes that have no added salt.

TOPPING IDEAS

• Mix together 2 tablespoons ricotta, 1 tablespoon chopped fresh chives or mint, and 1 tablespoon fresh basil. Add a little freshly squeezed lemon juice and season before spreading over 2 rice cakes.

• Blend together 2½ oz. pitted green olives with 1 garlic clove, 1 tablespoon extra virgin olive oil, and salt and pepper until you have a coarse pâté. Spread a little over 2 rice cakes.

• Arrange thin slices of ham or other cooked meat on top of 2 rice cakes. Halve a pear and remove the core from one half. Cut the cored half into thin slices and lay on top of the ham.

• Spread 1 tablespoon hummus over 2 rice cakes. Finely chop 2 slices of roasted red bell pepper and spoon on top of the rice cakes.

• Spread 1 tablespoon low-fat cream cheese over 2 rice cakes. Thinly slice 1 small, ripe fig and arrange on top of the rice cakes.

• Spread 1 tablespoon Quark over 2 rice cakes. Slice 3 strawberries and arrange on top of the rice cakes.

• Mix together 2 tablespoons cottage cheese with 1 finely chopped, pitted date in a bowl. Spoon the mixture on top of 2 rice cakes.

sardines and tomato on toast

Canned sardines are an ideal pantry standby, and are a good source of calcium, vitamin D, and long-chain omega-3 fatty acids—great brain food!

1 slice of whole-grain bread

reduced-fat mayonnaise, for spreading

2 oz. canned boneless, skinless sardines in olive oil, drained

1 small tomato, halved, seeded, and roughly chopped

a squeeze of fresh lemon juice

freshly ground black pepper

SERVES 1

Toast the bread on both sides, then lightly spread with the mayonnaise.

Put the sardines on top of the toast, then mash slightly with a fork. Arrange the tomato on top, then squeeze over a little lemon juice. Season with black pepper before serving.

Sardines and tuna

A Scottish study of more than 1,200 five-year-old children found that if their mothers ate fish once or more a week during pregnancy, they were less likely to have eczema than children of mothers who never ate fish. Eating fish weekly was also linked to a reduced risk of asthma among the mothers (*see* page 29).

oatcakes

These light, melt-in-the-mouth cookies are perfect served plain, or topped with a pure fruit spread, cottage cheese, or cooked ham for a more substantial snack. Oats and whole-wheat flour provide fiber, and oats contain low-GI carbohydrates, meaning they are absorbed slowly into the bloodstream and have a stabilizing effect on blood sugar levels.

¾ cup oat flour

1¼ cups whole-wheat flour, plus extra for dusting

2 teaspoons baking powder

¼ teaspoon sea salt

7 tablespoons butter, diced

1 tablespoon sugar

¼ cup low-fat milk

MAKES 24

2 baking sheets, lightly greased

Preheat the oven to 400°F.

Sift the oat flour, whole-wheat flour, and baking powder into a mixing bowl, adding any bran left in the strainer. Stir in the salt.

Rub the butter and sugar into the flour mixture using your fingertips until the mixture resembles bread crumbs. Pour in the milk and mix with a fork, then use your hands to form the mixture into a dough.

Turn the dough out onto a lightly floured work surface and knead briefly until smooth. Using a floured rolling pin, roll out the dough into a rectangle about 2 inches thick. Trim the edges and cut into 12 squares, re-rolling any trimmings as necessary.

Put the oatcakes on the prepared baking sheets and prick the top with a fork. Bake for 10 minutes until light golden, swapping the sheets halfway, if necessary, then transfer to a wire rack to cool.

VARIATIONS:

Apricot oatcakes
Finely chop 2 oz. unsulfured dried apricots or similar dried fruit and stir into the flour mixture in step 2. Continue to make the oatcakes following the instructions opposite.

Mixed seed oatcakes
Stir 2 tablespoons sunflower seeds into the flour mixture in step 2. Continue to make the oatcakes following the instructions opposite. Before placing the oatcakes on the baking sheets in step 5, sprinkle 2 teaspoons sesame seeds over the top and gently press them into the dough.

The ins and outs of fiber
Fiber is only found in plant foods—fruit, vegetables, breads and cereals (especially whole-grain types), nuts and seeds—and comes in two main forms. "Insoluble" fiber helps keep everything moving through the bowel and is best for preventing constipation (see page 25). Whole-grains and whole-wheat flour and breads, bran-based cereals, and most vegetables and fruits are the best sources. "Soluble fibre" is found in legumes, oats, barley, rye, and most fruits. Its gummy characteristics help to regulate the levels of cholesterol and glucose in your blood. Fiber can also keep bacteria in the bowel in balance.

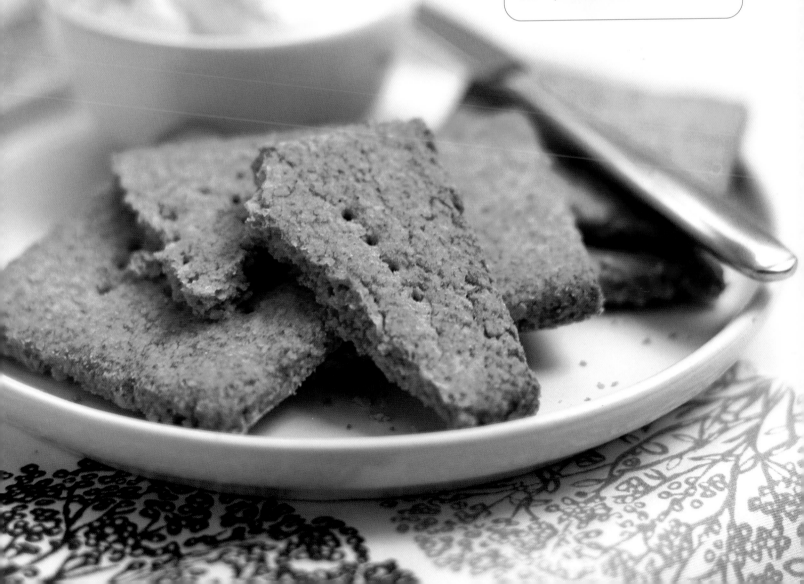

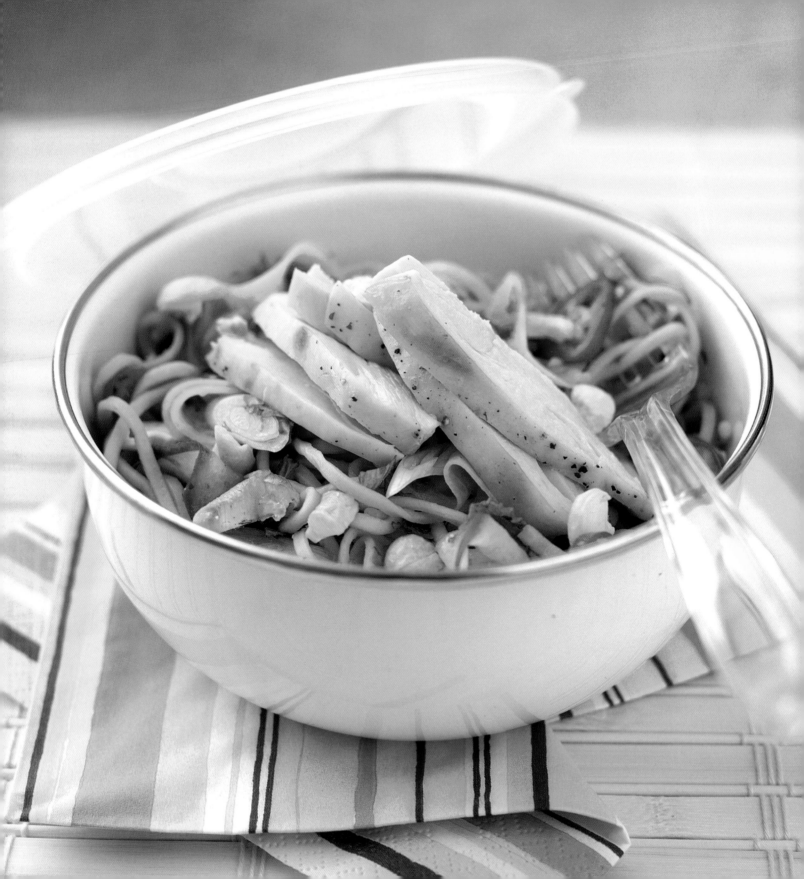

noodle box

This Thai-inspired salad makes a perfect addition to a lunchbox, as it will not wilt and is also nutritionally balanced. Make sure the chicken is cold before packing, and then store in a fridge or in an insulated lunchbox with an ice pack. Choose a firm, slightly unripe papaya for best results.

Preheat the broiler to high and line a broiler pan with foil. Broil the chicken breasts for 5–6 minutes each side until cooked through. Slice into strips and let cool.

Meanwhile, cook the noodles in plenty of boiling water following the instructions on the package, then drain. Refresh the noodles under cold running water, then leave in the colander. Mix together the ingredients for the dressing.

Using a vegetable peeler, shave the papaya lengthwise into ribbons. Repeat with the cucumber, discarding the seeds.

Put the cold noodles in a serving bowl and add the papaya, cucumber, scallions, herbs, and chile, if using. Pour the dressing over and toss until combined. Top with the strips of chicken and the toasted cashews.

2 skinless, boneless chicken breasts, about 6 oz. each

5 oz. medium egg noodles

1 firm papaya, halved, seeded, and peeled

5 inches cucumber, peeled

3 large scallions, thinly sliced diagonally

3 tablespoons chopped fresh mint

3 tablespoons chopped fresh cilantro

½ red chile, seeded and thinly sliced into rounds (optional)

2 tablespoons roughly chopped toasted cashews

DRESSING

1½ tablespoons freshly squeezed lime juice

1½ tablespoons Thai fish sauce

1½ tablespoons sugar

1 inch fresh ginger, peeled and grated

SERVES 2

summer gazpacho with crisp croutons

1 thick slice of day-old whole-grain bread, crusts removed

1½ lbs vine-ripened tomatoes

1 medium cucumber, cut lengthwise into quarters, seeded, and cut into chunks

1 large garlic clove, peeled and sliced

1 red bell pepper, seeded and roughly chopped

10 radishes, sliced

1 tablespoon extra virgin olive oil

2 tablespoons white wine vinegar

2 tablespoons freshly squeezed lemon juice

1 heaping teaspoon sun-dried tomato paste

sea salt and freshly ground black pepper

CROUTONS

1 tablespoon olive oil

2 thick slices of day-old wholemeal bread, crusts removed and cubed

TO SERVE

4 hard-cooked free-range eggs, quartered

16 pitted black olives, chopped

fresh basil leaves

SERVES 4

Full of the flavors of summer, this chilled soup is made up of antioxidant-rich salad ingredients. It will keep well in the fridge for a few days, and if you're looking for a light refreshment or a meal that is easy to manage when you're feeling queasy, a bowl of this makes a healthy snack. The serving suggestions can be left out if you are short of time, but they do add to the finished result.

Soak the bread in water until ready to use.

Make a small cross-shaped cut in the base of each tomato. Put the tomatoes in a heatproof bowl and cover with boiling water. Leave for 30 seconds, then peel, seed, and chop.

Tear the soaked bread into pieces and put half of it in a food processor with half of the tomatoes, cucumber, garlic, red bell pepper, radishes, olive oil, vinegar, lemon juice, sun-dried tomato paste, and ⅓ cup cold water. Process until puréed, then pour the soup into a pitcher.

Put the rest of the vegetables, olive oil, vinegar, lemon juice, sun-dried tomato paste, and ⅓ cup cold water in the food processor and process until chunky. If you like your soup smooth, purée all the ingredients with ⅔ cup cold water.

Combine the puréed vegetables and season with salt and pepper to taste. Cover and let chill in the fridge for about 2–3 hours.

Preheat the oven to 350°F. To make the croutons, put the oil in a small plastic bag and add the bread. Seal the bag and shake until the bread is coated in the oil. Put the bread cubes on a baking sheet and bake for 10–15 minutes until golden and crisp.

Pour the soup into 4 bowls and scatter over the croutons. Top with the quarters of hard-cooked egg and black olives. Garnish with basil leaves.

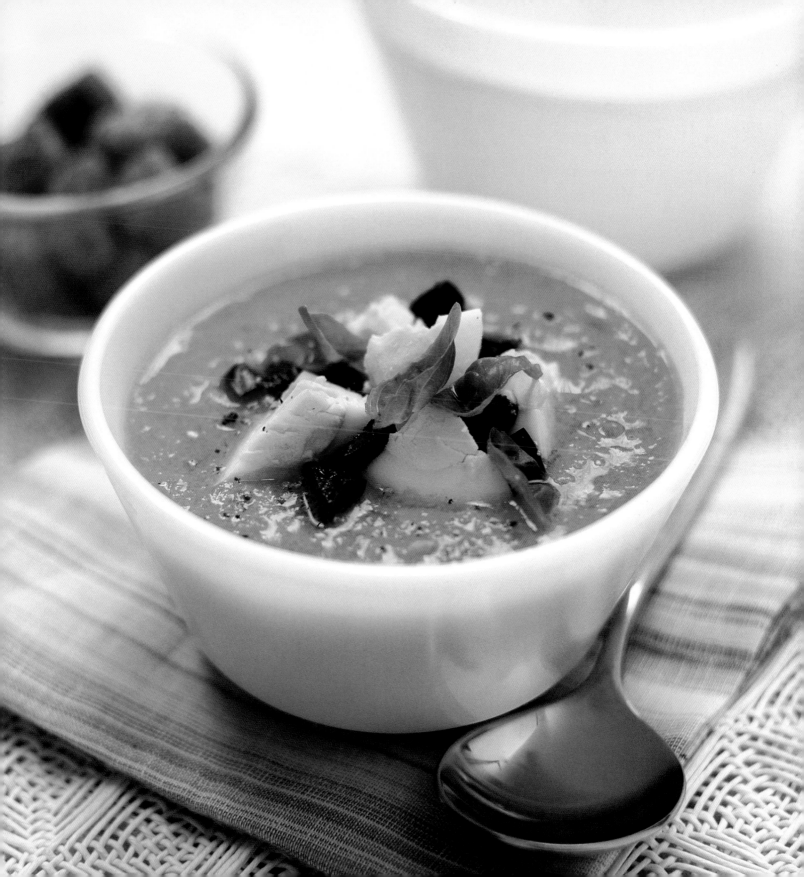

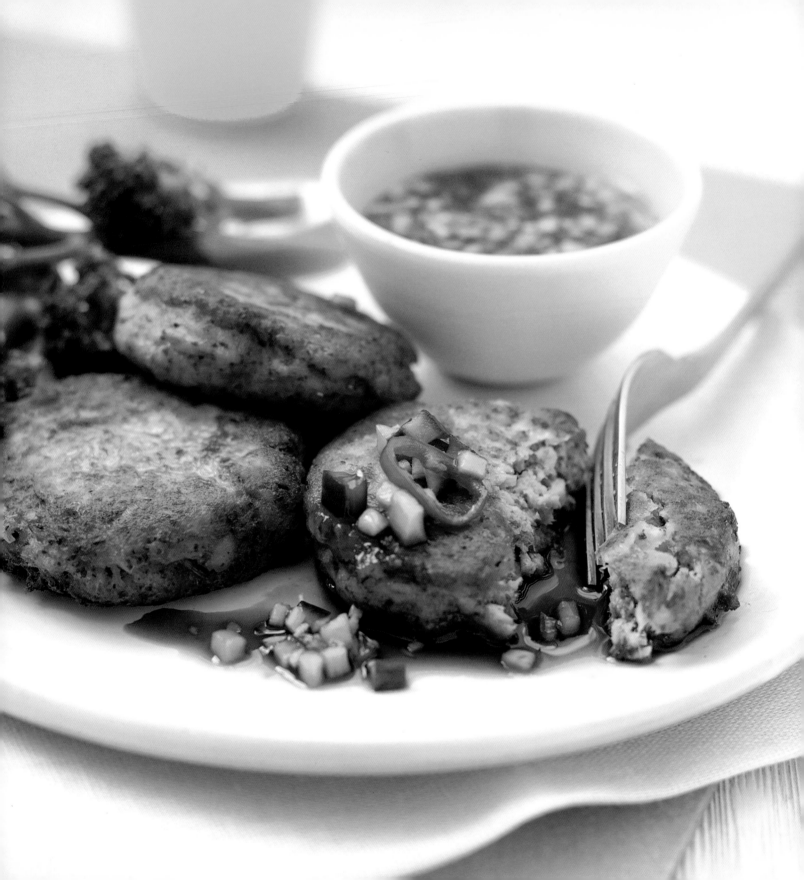

Thai salmon fishcakes with dipping sauce

Salmon is an excellent source of long-chain omega-3 fatty acids. For mothers-to-be, they are said to be particularly beneficial as they promote the healthy development of a baby's nervous system, eyes, and brain. For a more substantial lunch, serve the fishcakes with stir-fried or steamed green vegetables, salad, or noodles.

Put the scallions, hot pepper flakes, if using, cilantro, lime leaves, lemon grass, and eggs in a food processor and blend until finely chopped. Add the salmon, season with salt and pepper, and process briefly until the ingredients are combined; the mixture will be quite loose, but the cakes will hold together when cooked.

Heat 2 tablespoons oil in a large nonstick skillet. Put 2 tablespoons of the mixture per fishcake in the skillet—you will probably be able to cook 3–4 at a time. Fry the fishcakes for about 3 minutes until the bottom is set and golden, then carefully turn them over and cook for another 2–3 minutes.

Drain the fishcakes on paper towels and keep warm. Repeat to make about 12 fishcakes. Meanwhile, mix together the ingredients for the dipping sauce in a bowl.

Serve 3 fishcakes per person with a small bowl of the dipping sauce and wedges of fresh lime.

Note: The fishcakes can be frozen for up to 1 month. Let cool thoroughly, then stack, putting a piece of parchment paper between each cake, and wrap in plastic wrap.

4 scallions, sliced

½ teaspoon dried hot pepper flakes (optional)

a handful of chopped fresh cilantro

2 kaffir lime leaves, sliced

2 teaspoons finely chopped lemon grass

2 free-range eggs

14-oz. canned salmon, drained and skin and bones removed

sea salt and freshly ground black pepper

sunflower or canola oil, for frying

wedges of fresh lime, to serve

DIPPING SAUCE

3 inches cucumber, seeded and diced

1 inch fresh ginger, peeled and finely chopped

½ teaspoon light brown sugar

4 thin round slices of red chile (optional)

1 tablespoon Thai fish sauce

freshly squeezed juice of ½ lime

1 tablespoon soy sauce

MAKES ABOUT 12

SERVES 4

apple, watercress, and walnut salad

Apples and watercress make a nutritious partnership, with the final dish providing a wide range of vitamins, minerals, essential fatty acids, and phytochemicals. The walnuts provide protein and omega-3 fatty acids.

1 small red apple

2 oz. watercress

1 oz. walnuts, roughly chopped

Parmesan cheese shavings, to garnish

DRESSING

1 tablespoon extra virgin olive oil

1 tablespoon freshly squeezed lemon juice, plus extra for the apples

sea salt and freshly ground black pepper

SERVES 2

Quarter the apple, cut out the core, and slice thinly. Squeeze a little lemon juice over the apple to prevent it browning. Put the watercress in a large, shallow bowl, then add the apple and sprinkle with the walnuts.

Mix together the ingredients for the dressing, season to taste, and pour it over the salad. Toss the salad with your hands, then sprinkle with the Parmesan shavings. Serve with oatcakes or whole-wheat pita bread, if you like.

Watercress and similar greens

Watercress, arugula, cabbage, Brussels sprouts, broccoli, bok choy, kale, and cauliflower are all types of cruciferous vegetables. Their distinctive peppery taste is due to beneficial phytochemicals called "glucosinolates." Scientific studies link a regular intake of these to anti-cancer benefits. They also provide antioxidants, including vitamin C, as well as folic acid, beta-carotene (which the body converts to vitamin A), and minerals such as calcium.

crab and cilantro wrap

As well as tasty and convenient, canned crab is low in fat and a good source of protein, zinc, and selenium, making it particularly beneficial during pregnancy. Here, it is combined with vitamin C-rich yellow bell pepper and tangy lime juice, as well as cucumber and fresh cilantro, to make a light, nutritious filling for a soft tortilla wrap.

2 teaspoons reduced-fat mayonnaise

1 teaspoon freshly squeezed lime juice

1 large soft tortilla

2 oz. canned white crabmeat, drained

¼ yellow bell pepper, seeded, and cut into thin strips

1 inch cucumber, cut lengthwise into quarters, seeded, and cut into thin strips

1 heaping tablespoon chopped fresh cilantro

sea salt and freshly ground black pepper

SERVES 1

Mix together the mayonnaise and lime juice in a bowl.

Warm the tortilla in a dry skillet, then remove from the heat.

Spread the lime mayonnaise over the tortilla, then spoon the crabmeat down the center. Arrange the yellow bell pepper and cucumber over the top of the crab and sprinkle with the cilantro.

Season to taste, fold in the ends of the tortilla, then roll to encase the filling. Slice in half crosswise before serving.

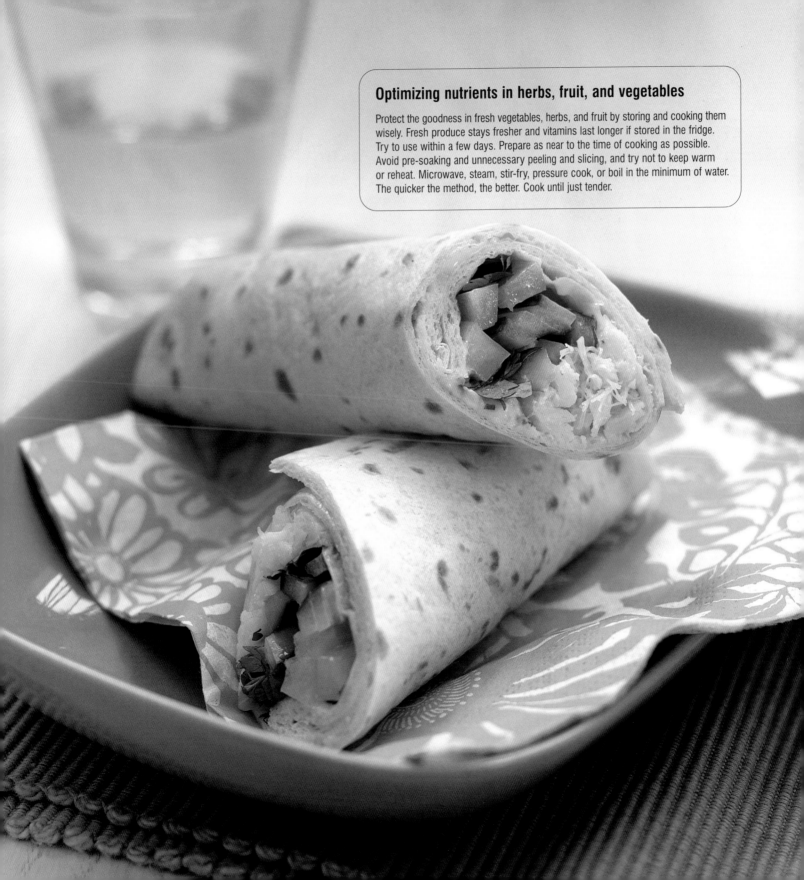

Optimizing nutrients in herbs, fruit, and vegetables

Protect the goodness in fresh vegetables, herbs, and fruit by storing and cooking them wisely. Fresh produce stays fresher and vitamins last longer if stored in the fridge. Try to use within a few days. Prepare as near to the time of cooking as possible. Avoid pre-soaking and unnecessary peeling and slicing, and try not to keep warm or reheat. Microwave, steam, stir-fry, pressure cook, or boil in the minimum of water. The quicker the method, the better. Cook until just tender.

fatoush

Fresh herbs add color, flavor, and nutritional value to this Lebanese salad, and although halloumi is not a traditional ingredient, the cheese adds valuable protein. This chunky salad is perfect in a lunchbox, but add the pita just before serving so it remains crisp.

1 large whole-wheat pita bread, opened out

1 small cucumber, cut lengthwise into quarters, seeded, and cut into chunks

2 large vine-ripened tomatoes, quartered, seeded, and cut into chunks

1 small red bell pepper, seeded and sliced

10 pitted black olives, halved

½ small red onion, cut into rings

3 tablespoons chopped fresh parsley

3 tablespoons chopped fresh mint

5 oz. halloumi cheese, patted dry and cut into cubes

DRESSING

2 tablespoons extra virgin olive oil, plus extra for frying

2 tablespoons freshly squeezed lemon juice

½ teaspoon ground cumin (optional)

sea salt and freshly ground black pepper

SERVES 2

Preheat the broiler to medium. Toast the pita bread until light golden and crisp. Let cool.

Meanwhile, mix together the ingredients for the dressing, leaving out the cumin, if preferred. Season with salt and pepper.

Put the cucumber, tomatoes, and red bell pepper in a serving bowl, then add the olives, onion, parsley, and mint. Pour the dressing over and toss until combined. Break the crisp pita into pieces and mix into the salad.

Heat a little oil in a skillet and fry the halloumi until it starts to color. Divide the salad between 2 plates, then top with the halloumi. (Let the halloumi cool if serving in a lunchbox.)

VARIATION
If in season, pomegranate seeds work well in this salad.

Calcium

Calcium is essential for building and maintaining healthy bones and teeth. A good intake is important throughout pregnancy, especially in the last 10 weeks when your baby's bones will be growing rapidly. The calcium-packed halloumi in this recipe means one serving provides around one-third of your recommended daily calcium intake.

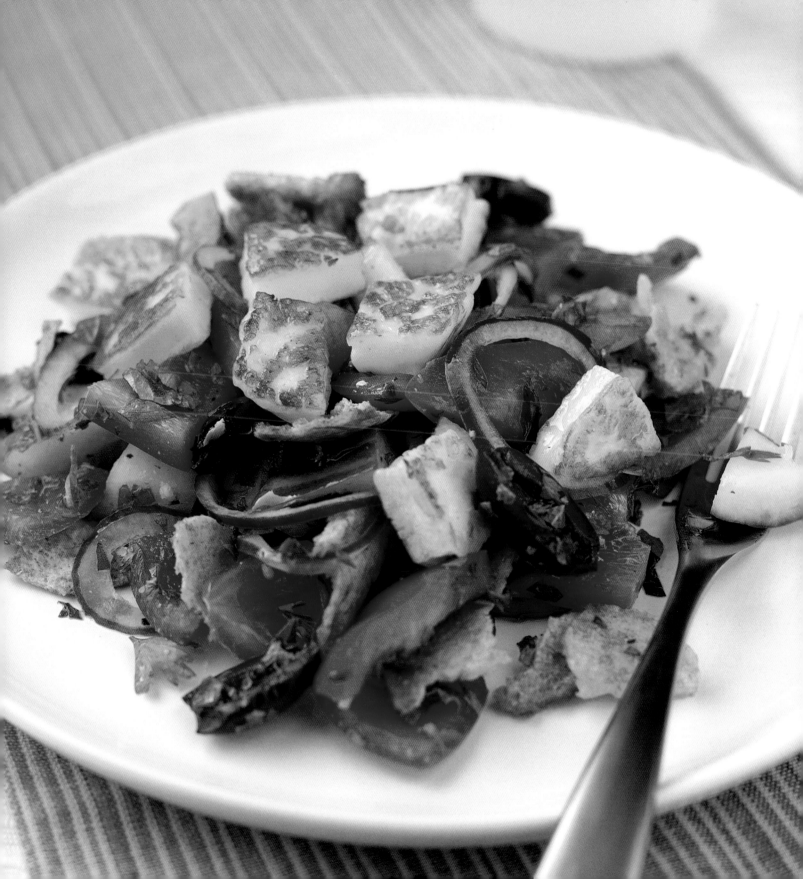

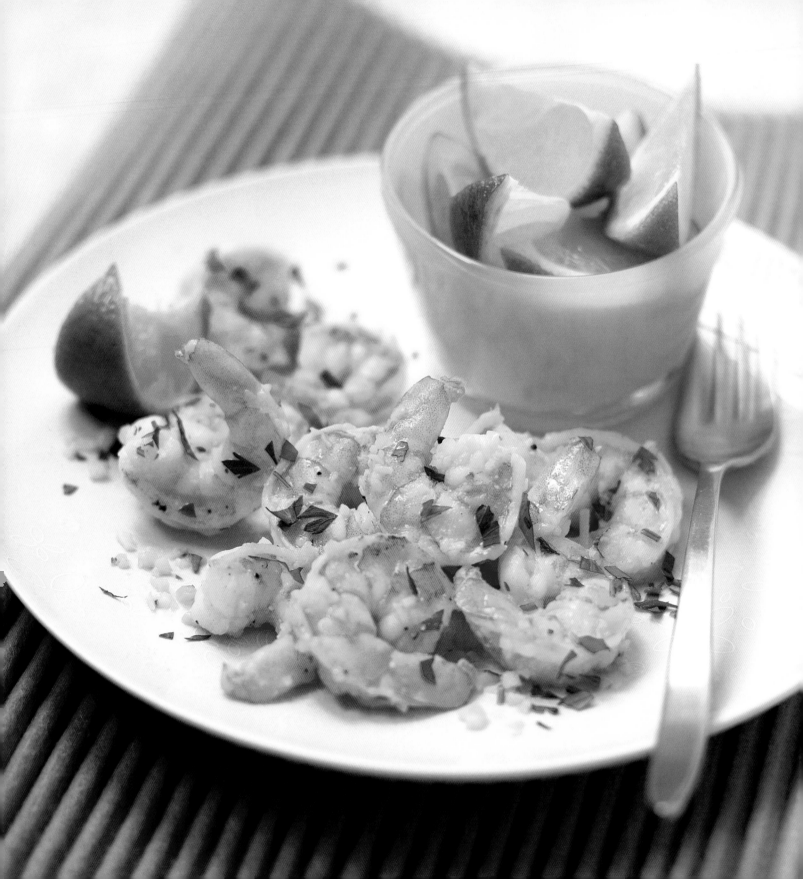

butterflied shrimp with garlic, lime, and ginger

12–14 oz. peeled uncooked large shrimp, tail on

2 tablespoons olive oil

2 inches fresh ginger, peeled and finely chopped

2 garlic cloves, finely chopped (optional)

freshly squeezed juice of 1 lime

sea salt and freshly ground black pepper

2 tablespoons chopped fresh parsley, to garnish

TO SERVE

1 lime, cut into wedges

SERVES 2

Ready to eat in a matter of minutes, this simple shrimp dish is full of zingy flavor and is light on the stomach. If you can't face garlic, it can be left out without adversely affecting the flavor of the finished result. Serve with a crisp mixed green salad and crusty bread to mop up the juices.

Make a slit down the curved back of each shrimp and scrape out the black vein, if there is one—this will also create the "butterflied" effect when the shrimp cook.

Heat the oil in a sauté pan over medium heat, add the shrimp, and fry, tossing them continuously, for 2 minutes. Add the ginger and garlic, if using, and continue to cook for another minute until the shrimp are pink. Add the lime juice and season well.

Put the shrimp in a serving dish and spoon over any juices from the pan. Garnish the shrimp with the parsley and serve with wedges of lime to squeeze over.

Shrimp and other shellfish

Like fish, these jewels from the sea brim with nutrients that are vital for you and your developing baby. Naturally low in fat, they provide protein, B vitamins, iodine, magnesium, selenium, zinc (oysters are the best source), and small amounts of long-chain omega-3 fatty acids. To avoid any risk of food poisoning, only eat thoroughly cooked or canned shellfish (*see* pages 27 and 29).

grilled vegetable salad with Parmesan

1½ tablespoons balsamic vinegar

1 tablespoon olive oil

1 large red onion, cut into
8 wedges

1 small red bell pepper, seeded and cut
into 6 wedges

1 small fennel bulb, trimmed and cut
into 6 wedges

10 asparagus spears, bases trimmed

2 zucchini, thinly sliced lengthwise

6 walnut halves, toasted and broken
into pieces

1 oz. Parmesan cheese

sea salt and freshly ground
black pepper

fresh basil leaves, to garnish

whole-wheat roll or bread, to serve

DIP

2 tablespoons reduced-fat mayonnaise

1 tablespoon green pesto

SERVES 2

a ridged stovetop grill pan

A warm salad made up of a nutritious combination of antioxidant-boosting vegetables and protein-rich nuts and cheese. The walnuts also provide omega-3 fatty acids. Grilling lends a wonderful barbecue flavor to vegetables, while retaining their crunchy texture; furthermore, this method of cooking does not require excessive amounts of oil.

Mix together the balsamic vinegar and oil in a shallow dish and add the vegetables. Turn the vegetables in the marinade until they are coated, then season with the salt and pepper.

Preheat a ridged stovetop grill pan. Arrange the onion, red bell pepper, and fennel in the pan and griddle for 7–8 minutes, turning halfway, until slightly charred and just tender.

Remove the onion, red pepper, and fennel from the grill pan and keep warm while you cook the rest of the vegetables. Arrange the asparagus and zucchini on the hot pan and griddle for 5–6 minutes, turning halfway.

While the vegetables are cooking, mix together the mayonnaise and pesto for the dip and set aside.

Arrange the vegetables on a serving platter and sprinkle over the walnuts. Using a vegetable peeler, slice the Parmesan into shavings, then scatter over the grilled vegetables with the basil leaves. Serve with the pesto dip and a fresh whole-wheat roll or bread.

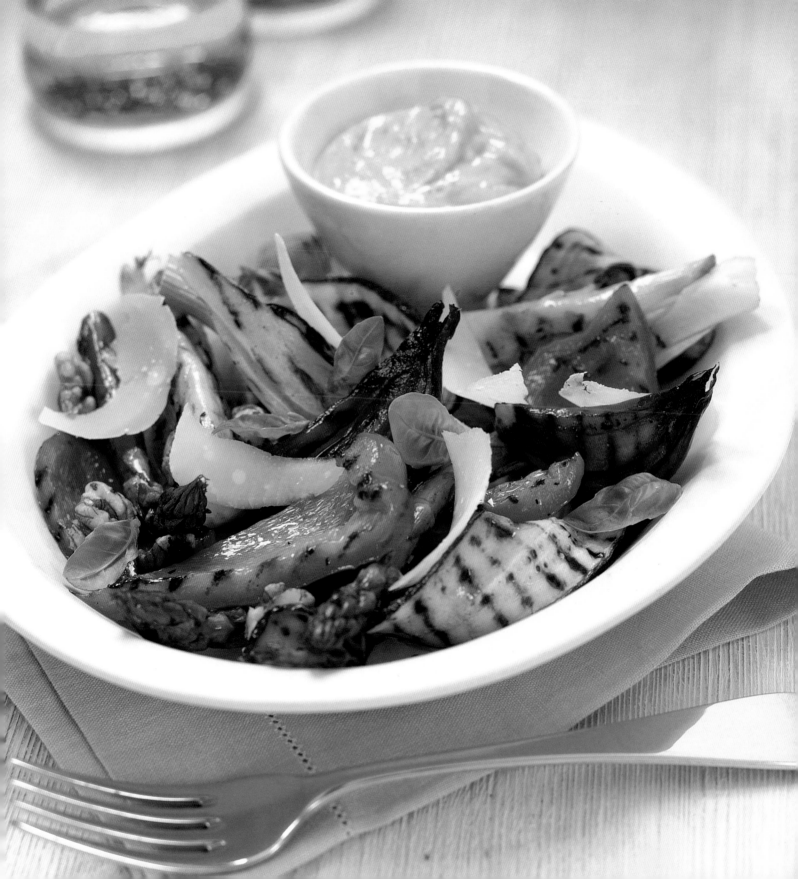

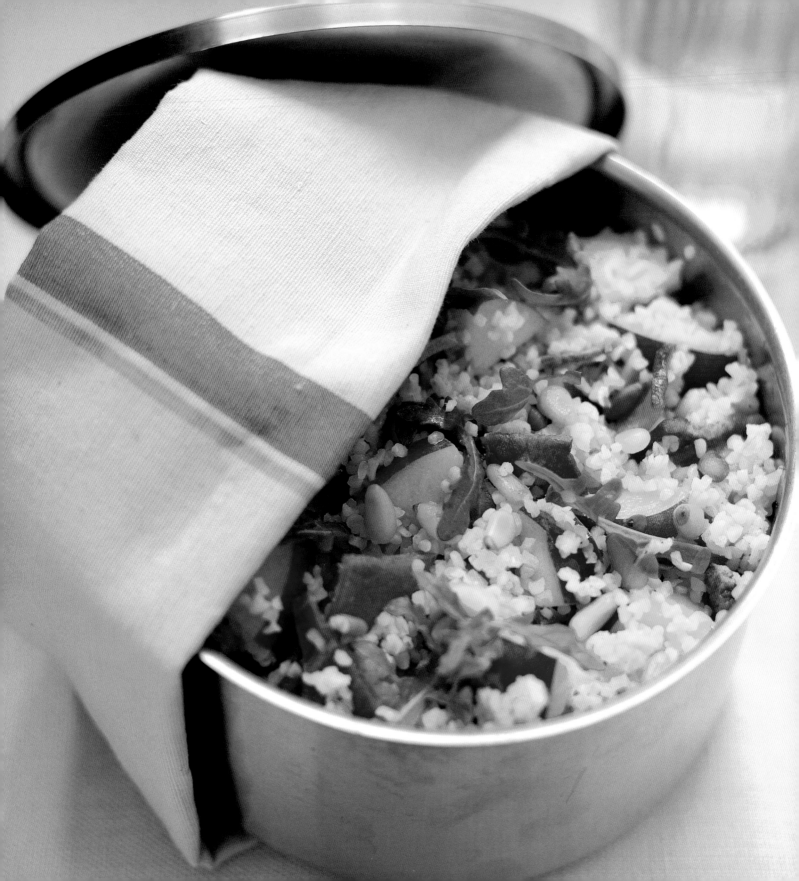

crispy bacon, arugula, and nectarine salad

Serve at room temperature rather than chilled to bring out the flavors of all the ingredients, particularly the nectarines.

½ cup bulgur wheat

3 slices lean bacon

1 nectarine, pitted and cut into bite-size chunks

a large handful of arugula leaves

2 tablespoons pine nuts, toasted (optional)

sea salt and freshly ground black pepper

DRESSING

1½ tablespoons extra virgin olive oil

1½ tablespoons freshly squeezed lemon juice

1 teaspoon Dijon mustard

SERVES 2

Preheat the broiler to high and line the broiler pan with foil.

Put the bulgur wheat in a saucepan and cover with water. Bring to a boil, then reduce the heat, cover with a lid and simmer for about 10 minutes until just tender. Drain well and put it in a shallow bowl.

Meanwhile, cook the bacon under the broiler until crisp. Remove from the broiler and let cool. Snip into ¾-inch lengths using scissors. Beat together the ingredients for the dressing.

Add the bacon, nectarine, and arugula to the bulgur wheat. Pour the dressing over and toss with your hands until everything is mixed together. Season well before sprinkling with the pine nuts, if using.

Note: If serving as part of a lunchbox, let the bulgur wheat and bacon cool thoroughly before putting in a lidded container.

vegetable, ham, and barley broth

This nurturing broth makes a nutritious light lunch, supper, or between-meal snack. It is filling enough to be served on its own, but if you are feeling particularly hungry, you could serve it with a slice of bread and calcium-rich cheese.

1 tablespoon sunflower or canola oil

2 onions, sliced

⅔ cup pearl barley, rinsed

1 celery rib, sliced

5 cups vegetable or chicken broth

2 bay leaves

1 bouquet garni

2 large carrots, peeled, halved lengthwise, and sliced

1 sweet potato, peeled and cut into bite-size chunks

7 oz. thickly cut cooked ham, diced, or ⅔ cup chickpeas, drained and rinsed

sea salt and freshly ground black pepper

SERVES 4

Heat the oil in a large saucepan and sauté the onions, half-covered, for 5 minutes. Add the barley and stir so that it is coated in the oil. Cook for another 2 minutes, stirring continuously.

Add the celery, broth, bay leaves, and bouquet garni to the pan. Bring to a boil, then reduce the heat and simmer, half-covered, for 30 minutes, occasionally skimming away any froth from the barley that rises to the surface.

Add the carrots, sweet potato, and ham and cook for another 15–20 minutes until the vegetables and barley are tender. Season to taste, then remove the bay leaves and bouquet garni before serving.

seared duck and pomegranate salad

During pregnancy, it is important to eat iron-rich foods daily, and duck, like red meat, is a particularly good source of this mineral. Duck also provides protein and B vitamins, while pomegranate offers high levels of antioxidants. Serve with warm whole-wheat pita.

1 tablespoon olive oil, plus a little extra for frying

5½ oz. mini skinless duck fillets

2 teaspoons clear honey

1 tablespoon soy sauce

2 oz. crisp salad greens, such as Bibb lettuce, shredded

1½ tablespoons freshly squeezed lemon juice

½ pomegranate, halved

2 tablespoons fresh cilantro leaves

sea salt and freshly ground black pepper

SERVES 2

Lightly brush a large nonstick skillet with oil. Heat the skillet, then add the duck fillets and sear for 3 minutes, turning halfway.

Mix together the honey and soy sauce and add to the skillet. Turn the duck to coat it in the sauce and fry for another 2 minutes until golden and the meat is cooked through. Remove the duck from the skillet and let cool slightly.

Arrange the salad greens in a shallow serving bowl. Mix together 1 tablespoon olive oil and the lemon juice, then pour it over the salad; toss it with your hands until the leaves are coated.

Arrange the duck on top of the salad greens. Remove the seeds from the pomegranate and sprinkle them over the salad, along with the cilantro leaves. Season to taste with salt and freshly ground black pepper.

Herbs

Different herbs add fresh flavors to food and can transform a humdrum dish into an appetizing delight. They also add beneficial antioxidants and small amounts of key nutrients. For example, mint contains omega-3 fatty acids, and parsley is great for vitamin C. In terms of safety, while care and advice must be taken with dried herbal preparations and remedies, using some fresh, everyday herbs in cooking is fine.

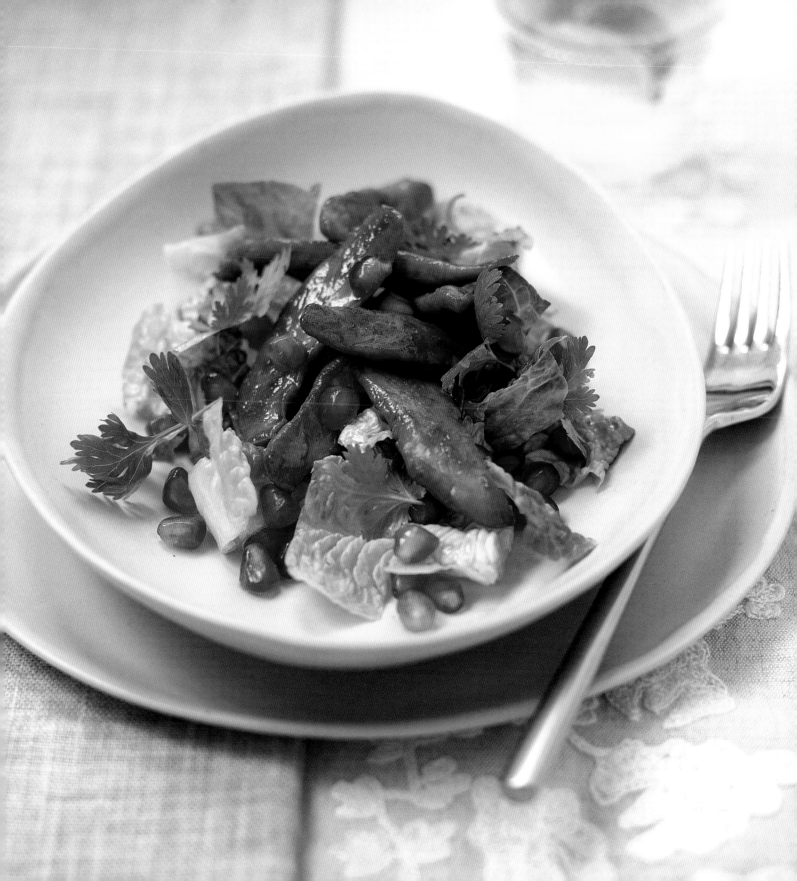

zucchini, potato, and onion tortilla

This light lunch checks all the right boxes. It contains everyday ingredients, is simple to make, and combines a balanced, sustaining combination of protein and carbohydrates. Serve with a watercress and tomato salad and crusty bread.

1¼ lbs potatoes, peeled and cut horizontally into 2-inch slices

2 tablespoons olive oil

2 onions, halved, then sliced into half-moon shapes

2 zucchini, diced

6 large free-range eggs

sea salt and freshly ground black pepper

SERVES 4–6

Cook the potatoes in boiling salted water for about 6 minutes until tender. Drain in a colander and cool under cold running water, then set aside.

Heat 1 tablespoon of the oil in a heavy-based nonstick skillet (about 13-inch diameter) with a heatproof handle over medium-low heat. Add the onions and sauté, covered, for 10 minutes, stirring frequently, until softened but not colored.

Add the zucchini and fry for another 3 minutes. Meanwhile, lightly beat the eggs in a large bowl and season to taste. Add the cooked onions, zucchini, and potatoes and turn until the vegetables are coated in the eggs.

Heat the remaining oil in the skillet. Remove the skillet from the heat and carefully pour the egg mixture into it. Make sure the vegetables are evenly distributed in the pan, pressing them down into the egg.

Preheat the broiler to medium.

Return the skillet to the hob and cook the tortilla for 6 minutes, until the bottom is set and slightly golden. To cook the top of the tortilla, put the skillet under the broiler and cook gently for 6–7 minutes, or until the egg is cooked.

Let the tortilla cool slightly before cutting into wedges.

golden tofu and vegetable wrap

Tofu is often underrated and underused, but when flavored well and cooked until golden and glossy, it is delicious. This meat alternative is packed with good-quality protein and provides omega-3 fatty acids.

6 oz. firm tofu, patted dry using paper towels and cut into 1½ x 1-inch strips

2 large soft tortillas

1 carrot, peeled and grated

½ red bell pepper, seeded and cut into thin strips

a handful of arugula leaves

sea salt and freshly ground black pepper

olive oil, for brushing

MARINADE

2 tablespoons soy sauce

1 tablespoon honey

1 tablespoon sweet chili sauce

2 tablespoons tomato ketchup

SERVES 2

a ridged stovetop grill pan

Mix together the ingredients for the marinade in a shallow dish. Add the tofu and spoon the marinade over until well covered. Cover and marinate for 1 hour.

Lightly brush a ridged stovetop grill pan with olive oil and heat until hot. Arrange the tofu in the pan and grill for 3 minutes each side until golden and it bears the marks of the pan.

Meanwhile, warm the tortillas—either wrap in foil and warm in the oven or warm in a dry skillet.

Put 2 pieces of tofu down the center of each tortilla and spoon over any remaining marinade. Divide the carrot, red bell pepper, and arugula between the tortillas, season to taste, then fold in the ends and sides of each tortilla to make a package. Cut each tortilla in half horizontally before serving.

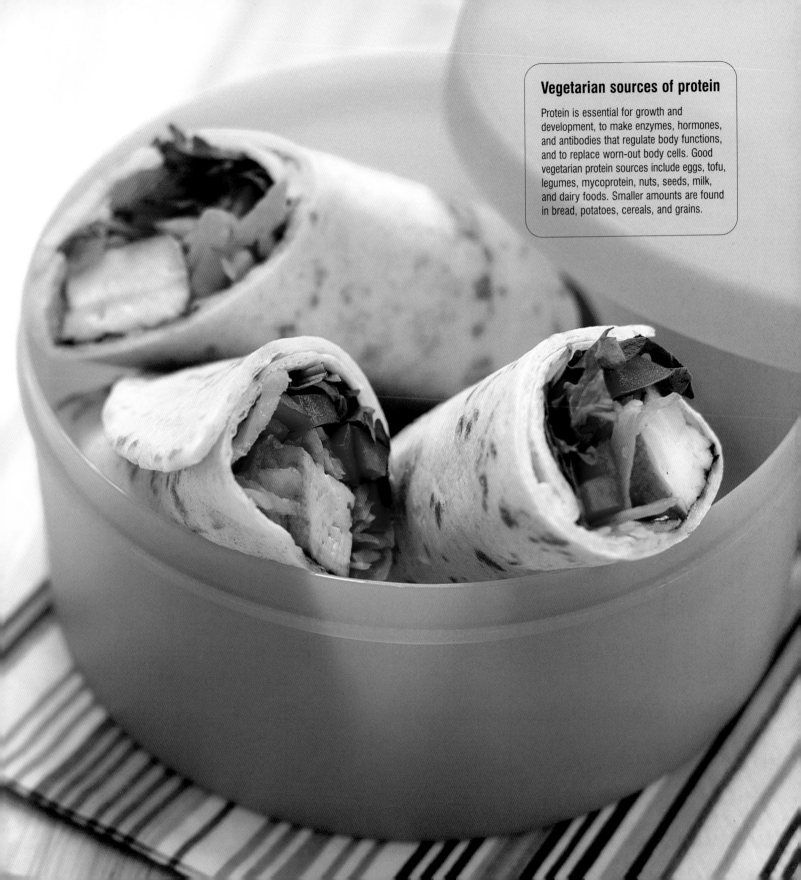

Vegetarian sources of protein

Protein is essential for growth and development, to make enzymes, hormones, and antibodies that regulate body functions, and to replace worn-out body cells. Good vegetarian protein sources include eggs, tofu, legumes, mycoprotein, nuts, seeds, milk, and dairy foods. Smaller amounts are found in bread, potatoes, cereals, and grains.

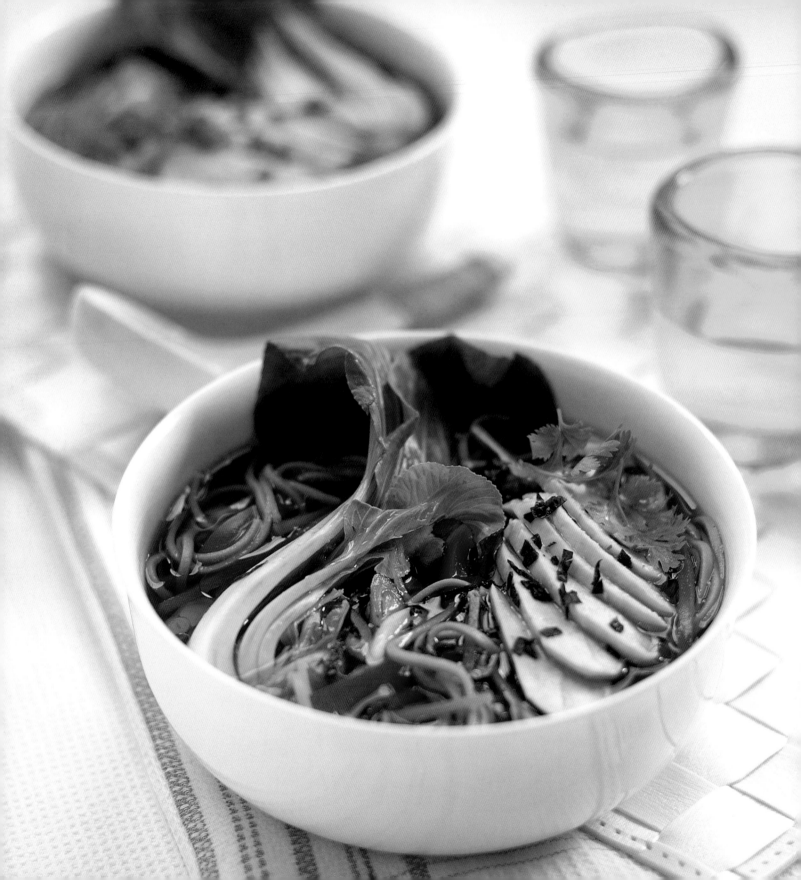

soba with chicken and vegetables

2 skinless, boneless chicken breasts, about 5 oz. each, sliced into thin strips, or 2 hard-cooked free-range eggs

3½ oz. soba noodles (buckwheat)

3 cups hot water

2 tablespoons brown rice miso paste

1 tablespoon soy sauce

1 inch fresh ginger, peeled and cut into thin strips

1 carrot, peeled, halved, and cut into thin strips

3 scallions, diagonally sliced

½ red bell pepper, seeded and cut into thin strips

2 baby bok choy, halved lengthwise

½ teaspoon toasted sesame oil

a sprinkling of toasted nori (seaweed) flakes

2 tablespoons fresh cilantro leaves

sunflower or canola oil, for brushing

SERVES 2

Don't be put off by the long list of ingredients—this Japanese-style soup couldn't be easier to make, and is light, soothing, and nourishing. It includes iodine-rich nori (a type of seaweed) and uses miso as its base (this healthy soya-bean paste is most often sold in health food shops).

Preheat the broiler to high and line the broiler pan with foil.

Arrange the chicken in the pan and brush with oil. Broil for 5–6 minutes each side until cooked through and there is no trace of pink in the center.

Meanwhile, cook the soba noodles in plenty of boiling water following the instructions on the package, then drain and refresh under cold running water. Set aside.

Put the hot water in a saucepan, add the miso paste, and stir until dissolved. Add the soy sauce, ginger, carrot, scallions, red bell pepper, and bok choy and bring up to boiling point. Reduce the heat and simmer for about 3 minutes until the bok choy is just tender. Stir in the sesame oil.

Divide the noodles between 2 shallow bowls and spoon over the vegetables and broth. Slice the chicken breasts and place on top, sprinkle with the nori and cilantro leaves, then serve.

Iodine

Iodine is needed for the thyroid gland to make hormones that regulate growth and metabolism (all the chemical processes in cells that enable our body to function). A lack of iodine during pregnancy can affect the development of your baby's brain. Iodine is also needed to help your baby start making his/her own thyroid hormones. Good sources include fish, shellfish, seaweed, dairy foods, and eggs. Vegans and vegetarians should make sure they have an adequate intake (see page 19).

hot smoked trout open sandwich
with avocado and beets

Inspired by the Scandinavian open sandwich, this version boasts a plethora of beneficial fats, such as long-chain omega-3 fatty acids (trout) and monounsaturated fat (avocado), along with cell- and skin-benefiting vitamin E.

1 small ciabatta loaf, halved lengthwise, then across, or 2–4 thick slices of light rye bread (depending on the size of the loaf)

1 teaspoon reduced-fat mayonnaise

2 teaspoons horseradish sauce

2 cooked beets in natural juice, thinly sliced into rounds

2 hot smoked trout fillets, about 4 oz. total weight

a squeeze of fresh lemon juice

1 small avocado, pitted, peeled, and thinly sliced

sea salt and freshly ground black pepper

a few sprigs of fresh dill, to garnish (optional)

SERVES 2

a ridged stovetop grill pan

Grill or lightly toast the bread. Meanwhile, mix together the mayonnaise and horseradish, and spread over the bread once toasted.

Arrange the sliced beets over the bread in a single layer, then put the trout fillets on top. Squeeze a little lemon juice over the avocado to prevent it browning and arrange on top of the trout.

Season well to taste and garnish with a few sprigs of dill, if using.

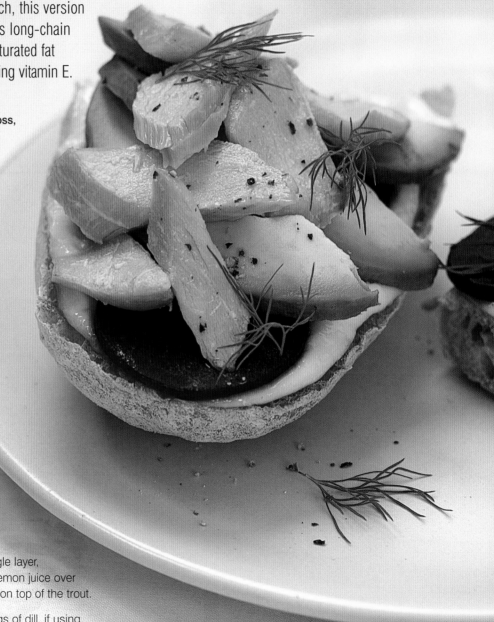

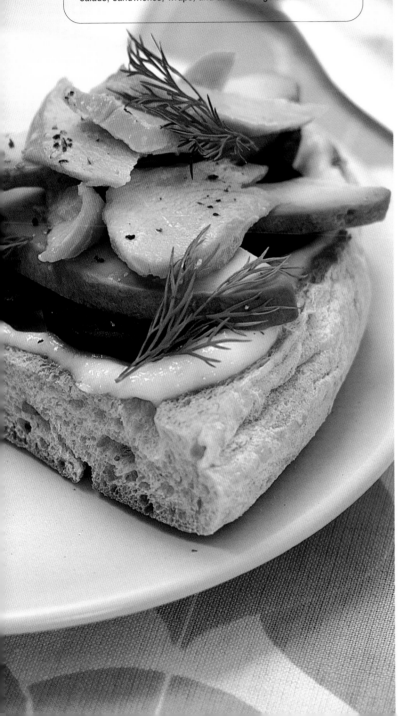

Beets

Beets, whether freshly grated or cooked (but not pickled), are a great source of folic acid, vital for the normal development of your baby's spinal cord (*see* page 15–16). Enjoy beets in salads, sandwiches, wraps, and as a hot vegetable.

Italian white bean and rosemary soup

Soothing and restorative, this soup is just right if you crave something light, yet warming and nutritious. A small bowlful also makes a sustaining snack, thanks to nutritious beans brimming with slow release energy.

1 tablespoon olive oil, plus extra for drizzling

2 onions, roughly chopped

2 large carrots, peeled and sliced

1 celery rib, sliced

14-oz. can cannellini beans, drained and rinsed

14-oz. can butter beans, drained and rinsed

2 x 4-inch sprigs of fresh rosemary

1 bouquet garni

3 cups vegetable or chicken broth

sea salt and freshly ground black pepper

TO SERVE (PER PERSON)

2 breadsticks

2 slices of thinly cut cooked ham

2 teaspoons red pesto

SERVES 3–4

Heat the oil in a large saucepan with a lid. Add the onions and sauté over medium heat, half-covered, for 5 minutes until softened. Toss in the carrots and celery, stir to coat the vegetables in the oil, and sauté, half-covered, for another 2 minutes. Stir in the cannellini beans, butter beans, rosemary, and bouquet garni, then pour in the broth.

Bring to a boil, then reduce the heat, half-cover the pan, and simmer over medium-low heat for 20 minutes until the vegetables are tender. Stir the soup occasionally during cooking.

Take the pan off the heat and remove the rosemary and bouquet garni. Using a hand-held blender, purée the soup until smooth and creamy. Season to taste with salt and freshly ground black pepper. To serve, wrap each breadstick in a slice of ham. Ladle the soup into bowls and top each one with 2 teaspoons red pesto and a drizzle of olive oil; accompany with the breadsticks.

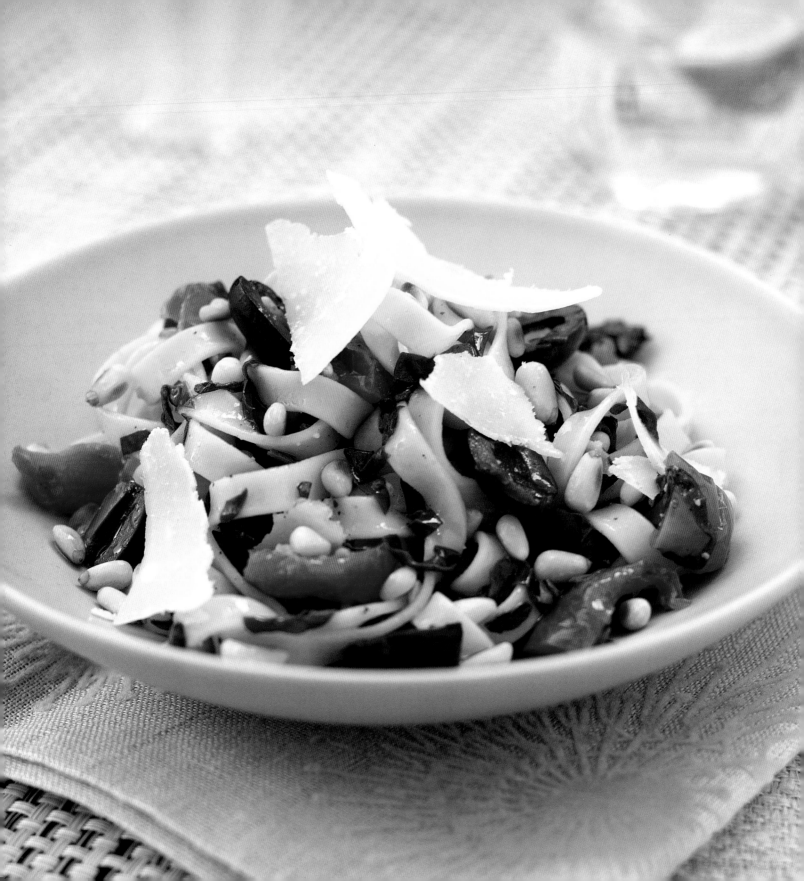

tagliatelle with half-dried tomatoes and toasted pine nuts

2 tablespoons pine nuts

6½ oz. dried tagliatelle

2 tablespoons olive oil

2 garlic cloves, finely chopped

3½ oz. half-dried tomatoes in oil (or marinated in oil, garlic, and oregano), roughly chopped

4 oz. fresh spinach, stalks removed and leaves thinly sliced

10 pitted black olives, halved

sea salt and freshly ground black pepper

Parmesan cheese shavings, to serve

SERVES 2

Satisfyingly quick to make and light to eat, the vitamin C in this dish will help the absorption of the iron found in the spinach.

Put the pine nuts in a dry skillet and toast for a few minutes, turning occasionally, until light golden—keep an eye on them, as they burn easily.

Bring a large saucepan of salted water to a boil. Cook the pasta following the instructions on the package until al dente. Drain, reserving ½ cup of the cooking water.

Heat the olive oil in a skillet and add the garlic, tomatoes, and spinach. Fry, stirring continuously, for 2–3 minutes until the spinach has wilted.

Add the olives, pasta, and reserved cooking water. Season well and toss thoroughly over low heat until heated through and combined.

Transfer to 2 plates and serve sprinkled with the Parmesan shavings, and salt and pepper to taste.

Phytochemicals and antioxidants

Phytochemicals are natural compounds found in plant foods that give them their distinctive taste and color. These protect our health in different ways. Many are antioxidants, which defend against damage to healthy body cells. Different colors reflect the presence of different phytochemicals and antioxidants—so to make the most of your fruit and vegetables, enjoy a rainbow of colors every day. The ingredients in this easy pasta dish get you off to a great start.

honey-glazed salmon
with grilled asparagus

This dish is packed with folic acid and long-chain omega-3 fatty acids, both vital for a healthy pregnancy. It's also simple enough for a quick supper, or would make a fantastic dinner party dish served with noodles or new potatoes.

2 salmon fillets, about 6 oz. each

10 asparagus spears, bases trimmed

olive oil, for brushing

2 teaspoons toasted sesame seeds, to serve

MARINADE

1 garlic clove, sliced (optional)

2 tablespoons soy sauce

2 tablespoons honey

2 teaspoons toasted sesame oil

1 teaspoon balsamic vinegar

SERVES 2–4

a ridged stovetop grill pan

Mix together the ingredients for the marinade in a shallow non-metallic dish. Put the salmon, skin-side up, in the dish and spoon the marinade over. Cover and marinate in the fridge for at least 1 hour.

Preheat the broiler to high. Line a broiler pan with foil and put the salmon, skin-side up, on top, reserving the marinade. Broil for 3–4 minutes, then turn the fish and spoon over some of the marinade. Cook for another 3 minutes until the tops of the fillets are golden and the fish is cooked.

Meanwhile, heat the stovetop grill pan and brush the asparagus with oil. Arrange the asparagus in the pan and cook for 4–5 minutes until tender.

Put the remaining marinade in a small saucepan and bring up to boiling point, then reduce the heat and cook until slightly thickened and reduced.

Arrange the asparagus on 2 plates, then top with the salmon. Spoon the marinade over the fish and sprinkle with the sesame seeds.

Folic acid and omega-3 fats

Salmon is great for long-chain omega-3 fatty acids (*see* page 17), while the asparagus is a fantastic folic acid booster. Both are vital, but getting enough folic acid is especially important during the first 12 weeks of pregnancy, when your baby's spinal cord is forming. A good intake of omega-3 becomes even more vital during the last 12 weeks of your pregnancy, when your baby's brain has a growth spurt.

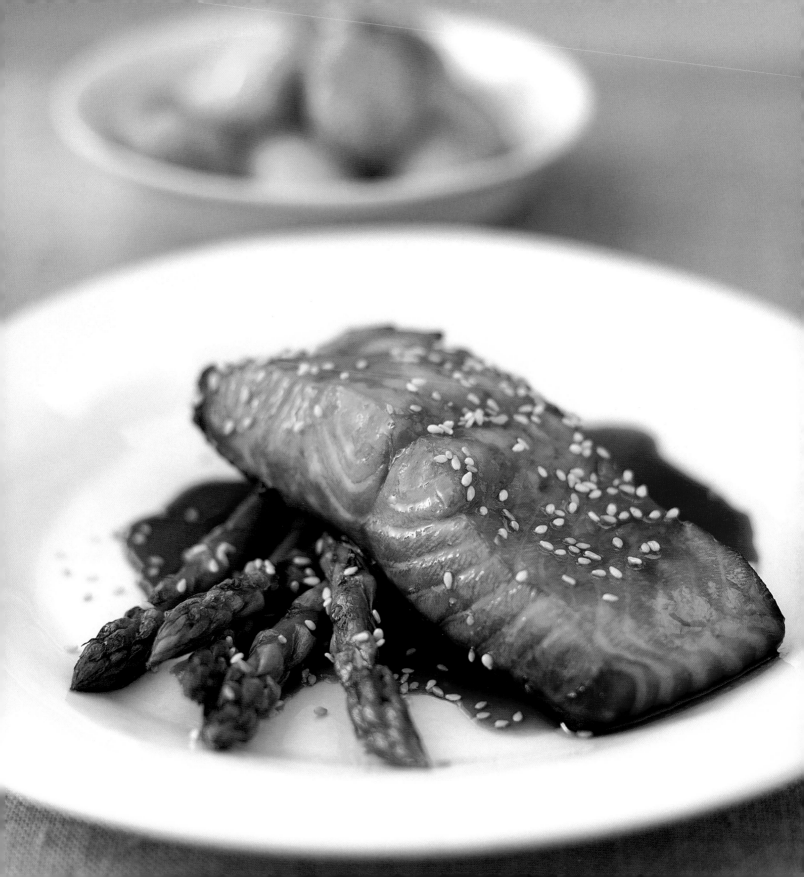

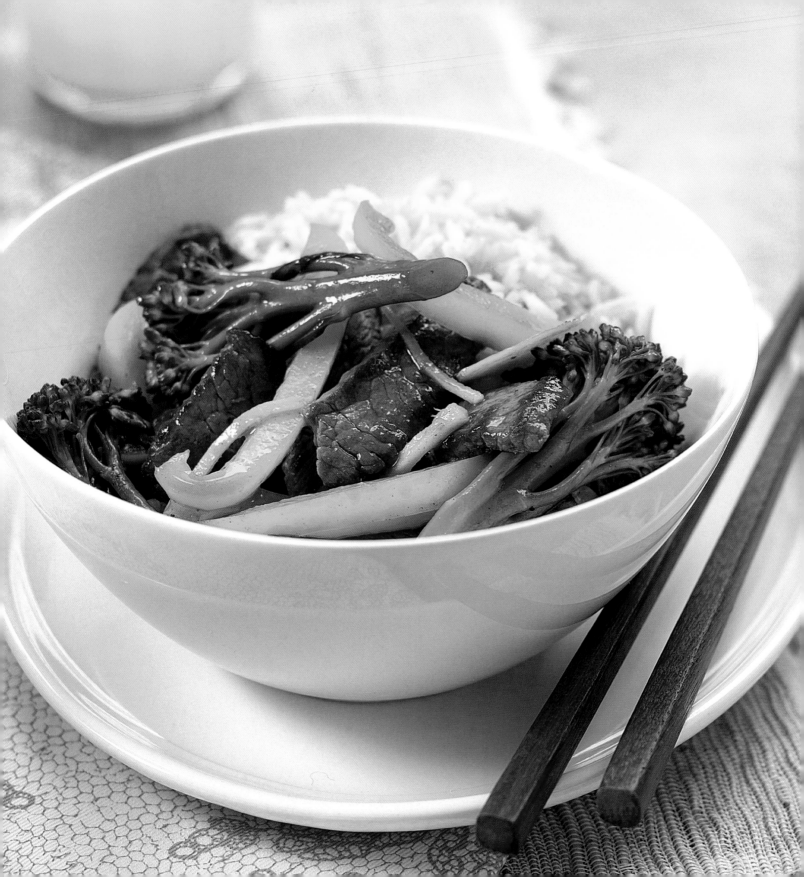

beef and broccolini stir-fry

Anemia is not unusual in pregnancy, so it is vital to eat adequate amounts of iron-rich foods. Red meat, such as beef, provides plentiful amounts in an easily absorbable form. All types of broccoli are nutritional powerhouses, providing folic acid along with many other vitamins and minerals. Serve this colorful stir-fry with noodles or brown rice.

6 oz. broccolini, stalks diagonally sliced

1 tablespoon peanut or canola oil

8 oz. lean beef sirloin, thinly sliced across the grain

1 yellow bell pepper, seeded and sliced

2 garlic cloves, sliced

1 inch fresh ginger, peeled and cut into thin matchsticks

3 tablespoons fresh orange juice (not from concentrate)

1–1½ tablespoons soy sauce

1 teaspoon toasted sesame oil

freshly ground black pepper

SERVES 2

Steam the broccolini for 2 minutes, then refresh under cold running water.

Heat a wok until hot. Add the peanut oil, then add the beef and stir-fry for 1–2 minutes until browned. Remove the beef from the wok using a slotted spoon and set aside.

Put the broccolini, yellow bell pepper, garlic, and ginger in the wok and stir-fry for 2 minutes. Return the beef to the pan, stir, then pour in the orange juice, soy sauce, and sesame oil and stir-fry for another minute.

Season with freshly ground black pepper and serve.

simple poached chicken with vegetables

This quick, light, and satisfying supper is easy on the digestive system and offers a nutritious combination of antioxidants, provided by the vegetables, and low-fat protein from the chicken. Serve with new potatoes.

1⅔ cups chicken broth

2 bay leaves

1 bouquet garni

3–4 sprigs of fresh thyme, plus extra to garnish (optional)

2 skinless, boneless chicken breasts, about 11 oz. total weight

1 large leek, diagonally sliced

2 carrots, peeled and diagonally sliced

2 zucchini, diagonally sliced

2 teaspoons unsalted butter

sea salt and freshly ground black pepper

SERVES 2

Put the broth, bay leaves, bouquet garni, and thyme in a large sauté pan and bring up to boiling point. Reduce the heat and put the chicken breasts in the pan, then cover with a lid and simmer for 10 minutes.

Add the leek and carrots to the pan and press them down to submerge them in the broth. Simmer, covered, for 8 minutes. Stir in the zucchini and cook for another 5 minutes, or until the chicken is cooked (there should be no trace of pink in the center) and the vegetables are tender.

Using a slotted spoon, remove the chicken and vegetables. Divide the chicken and vegetables between 2 shallow bowls. Cut the chicken into thick slices.

Remove the bay leaves and bouquet garni and discard. Pour off all but ⅔ cup of the chicken broth and add the butter. Warm through, stirring, until the sauce has reduced slightly. Season to taste.

Pour the sauce over the chicken and vegetables before serving, and garnish with extra thyme, if liked.

turkey and bay skewers
with potato, olive, and tomato salad

1 tablespoon olive oil

1 tablespoon freshly squeezed lemon juice

12 small fresh bay leaves

1 small unwaxed lemon, halved and cut into 12 small wedges

10 oz. skinless, boneless turkey breast, cut into 12 large bite-size chunks

sea salt and freshly ground black pepper

POTATO, OLIVE, AND TOMATO SALAD

14 oz. new potatoes, scrubbed

12 pitted black olives, quartered

2 vine-ripened tomatoes, seeded and cut into chunks

3 tablespoons chopped fresh flat-leaf parsley

a handful of fresh basil leaves

1½ tablespoons freshly squeezed lemon juice

1½ tablespoons extra virgin olive oil

SERVES 2

4 wooden (see method) or metal skewers

These turkey kebabs are infused with the flavor of lemon and bay leaves and provide a low-fat source of protein, selenium and B vitamins.

If using wooden skewers, soak in water for 30 minutes to prevent them burning during cooking. Alternatively, use metal skewers.

Preheat the broiler to medium-high and line a broiler pan with foil.

To make the potato salad, cook the potatoes in boiling water for 12 minutes, or until tender. Drain and let cool slightly. Halve or quarter the potatoes if large, then put in a salad bowl with the olives, tomatoes, parsley, and basil leaves. Mix together the lemon juice and olive oil and pour over the salad. Season to taste and toss until everything is combined.

To make the skewers, mix together the olive oil and lemon juice.

To assemble the skewers, follow this order of ingredients for each one: bay leaf, lemon, turkey, lemon, turkey, bay leaf, lemon, turkey, bay leaf.

Arrange the 4 skewers in the broiler pan. Brush with the olive oil and lemon juice mixture and broil for 4 minutes. Turn the skewers, brush with more of the olive oil and lemon juice, and broil for another 3–5 minutes, or until the turkey is cooked through.

Serve the turkey skewers with a helping of the potato salad.

Poultry

Poultry, which includes chicken, turkey, and duck, is a tasty and versatile source of protein, minerals, and B vitamins. While higher in fat, the darker meat tends to contain more iron, zinc, and selenium, so enjoy some of both. The skin is the fattiest part, so avoid whenever possible, and trim off any fat. Ensure poultry is cooked right through and no pinkness remains.

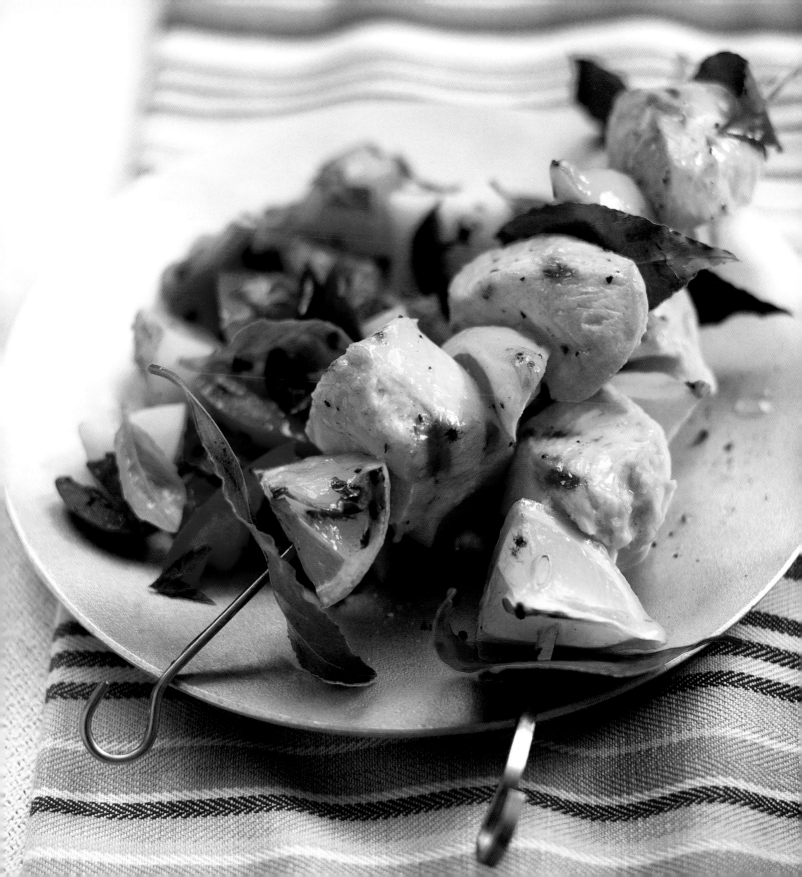

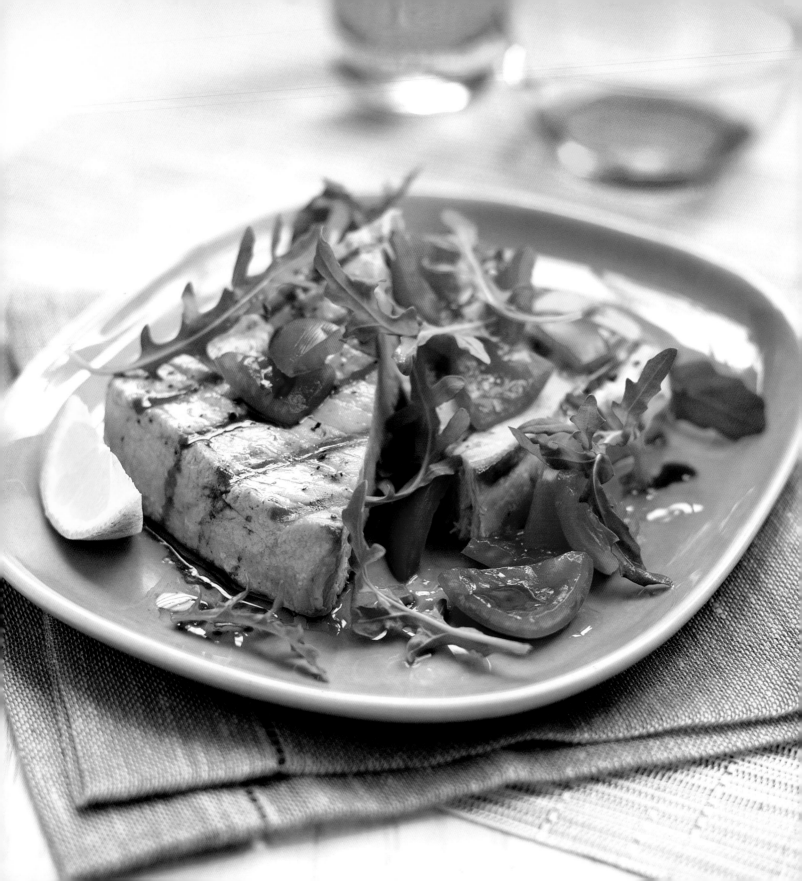

grilled tuna with arugula and tomatoes

A great summer supper dish, this warm salad just needs the addition of new potatoes or crusty bread. It is important to include a range of essential fatty acids in your diet, and tuna provides long-chain omega-3, essential for your baby's healthy eye, nerve, and brain development.

1½ tablespoons extra virgin olive oil

1½ tablespoons balsamic vinegar

2 thick tuna steaks, about 6 oz. each

5 vine-ripened tomatoes, halved, seeded, and cut into chunks

a large handful of arugula leaves

a squeeze of fresh lemon juice

sea salt and freshly ground black pepper

SERVES 2

a ridged stovetop grill pan

Mix together the olive oil and balsamic vinegar and lightly brush some of the mixture over the tuna steaks.

Heat a stovetop grill pan until very hot. Put the tuna in the pan and cook for about 2 minutes each side until slightly charred on the outside and just cooked on the inside.

Place the tuna on 2 serving plates and slice in half. Scatter the tomatoes and rocket around the tuna. Squeeze over a little lemon juice, and drizzle with the olive oil and balsamic dressing. Season to taste with salt and pepper.

Vegetables and salad

Naturally low in fat and calories and brimming with antioxidants, phytochemicals (see pages 12–13), vitamins, and minerals, vegetables of all types are a vital part of a healthy diet. It's easy to get stuck on old favorites, but the wider the variety of types and colors you enjoy each week, the more you optimize their health benefits. Aim to make some salad or vegetables part of lunch and dinner (use the recipes for inspiration), and try vegetable-based soups or raw veggie sticks as snacks.

dahl with baked fish

The lentil is much underrated, but this low-fat, protein-rich legume provides iron, folic acid, and zinc as well as fiber.

2 tablespoons sunflower or canola oil

1 large onion, chopped

2 large garlic cloves, peeled and crushed

4 green cardamom pods, split

2 bay leaves

2 carrots, peeled and grated

2 tablespoons grated fresh ginger

2 teaspoons ground coriander

½–1 teaspoon ground red chili

1 cup red split lentils

¾ cup canned reduced-fat coconut milk

¾ cup tomato passata or purée

2 teaspoons garam masala

freshly squeezed juice of 1½ limes

4 thick white fish fillets, about 6 oz. each

¼ cup chopped fresh cilantro, plus extra to garnish

2 teaspoons cumin seeds

2 teaspoons mustard seeds

sea salt and freshly ground black pepper

SERVES 4

Preheat the oven to 400°F. Heat 1 tablespoon of the oil in a large heavy-based saucepan and sauté the onion for 10 minutes until softened. Add the garlic and sauté for 30 seconds, stirring, followed by the cardamom, bay leaves, carrots, ginger, and ground spices. After a minute, add the lentils, 2 cups water, the coconut milk, and passata to the pan, stir, and bring to a boil, then reduce the heat and simmer, covered, for 20 minutes. Stir the garam masala and the juice of 1 lime into the lentil mixture and cook, covered, for 20 minutes. Stir occasionally.

Meanwhile, brush a large piece of foil with a little of the remaining oil. Lay the fish on top, season, squeeze over the remaining lime juice, then fold over the foil to make a package, put on a baking sheet and cook in the oven for 20 minutes, or until the fish is just cooked. When the lentils are tender, remove the pan from the heat and purée with a hand-held blender until smooth, or leave it chunky. Stir in the fresh cilantro and season. Heat the remaining oil in a small skillet and add the cumin and mustard seeds. Toss in the skillet for 30 seconds until they pop and smell toasted, then remove from the heat. Divide the dahl between 4 shallow bowls, and top with the fish. Sprinkle with the spices and cilantro.

linguine with shrimp, peas, and zucchini

This easy and revitalizing pasta dish is packed with protein, zinc, folic acid, and other B vitamins.

6½ oz. dried linguine

2 zucchini, sliced

1 cup frozen baby peas

1 tablespoon olive oil

1 large garlic clove, finely chopped (optional)

6½ oz. cooked, shelled, deveined large shrimp

zest of ½ unwaxed lemon

2 tablespoons freshly squeezed lemon juice

2 tablespoons reduced-fat sour cream

sea salt and freshly ground black pepper

fresh basil leaves, to garnish

SERVES 2

Cook the pasta in plenty of boiling salted water following the instructions on the package until al dente. Drain the pasta, reserving ¼ cup of the cooking water.

Meanwhile, steam the zucchini and baby peas until cooked.

While the pasta and vegetables are cooking, heat the olive oil in a heavy-based saucepan and fry the garlic, if using, over medium-low heat for 1 minute. Add the shrimp, lemon zest and juice, sour cream, and reserved cooking water. Cook, stirring, for about 1 minute until the shrimp are heated through.

Add the pasta, zucchini, and baby peas and toss until the ingredients are combined and warmed through. Season to taste and serve sprinkled with basil leaves.

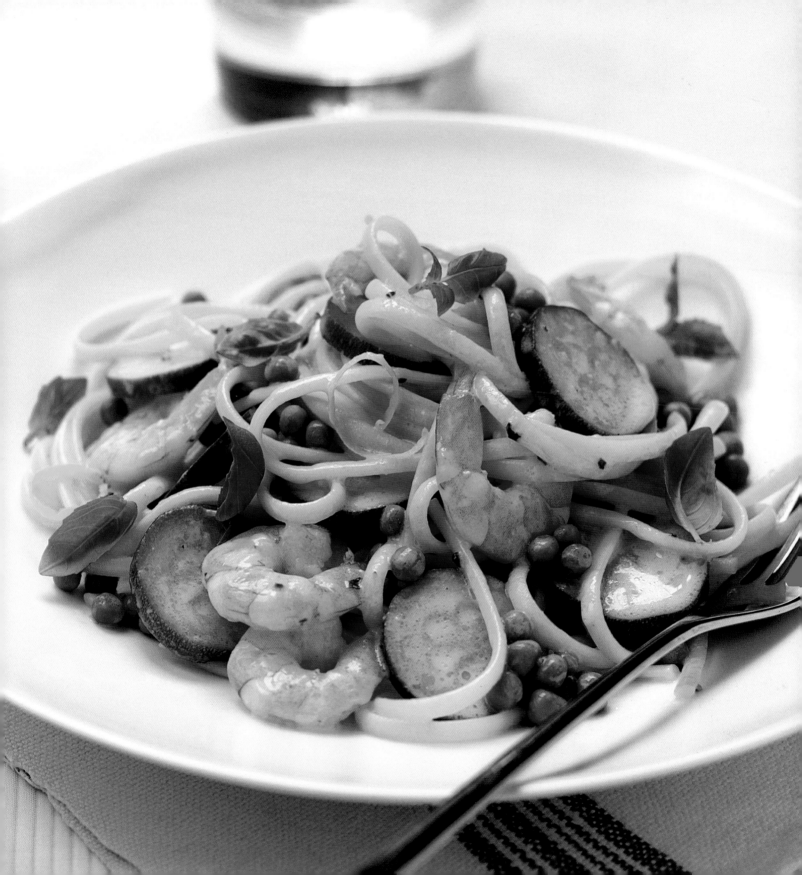

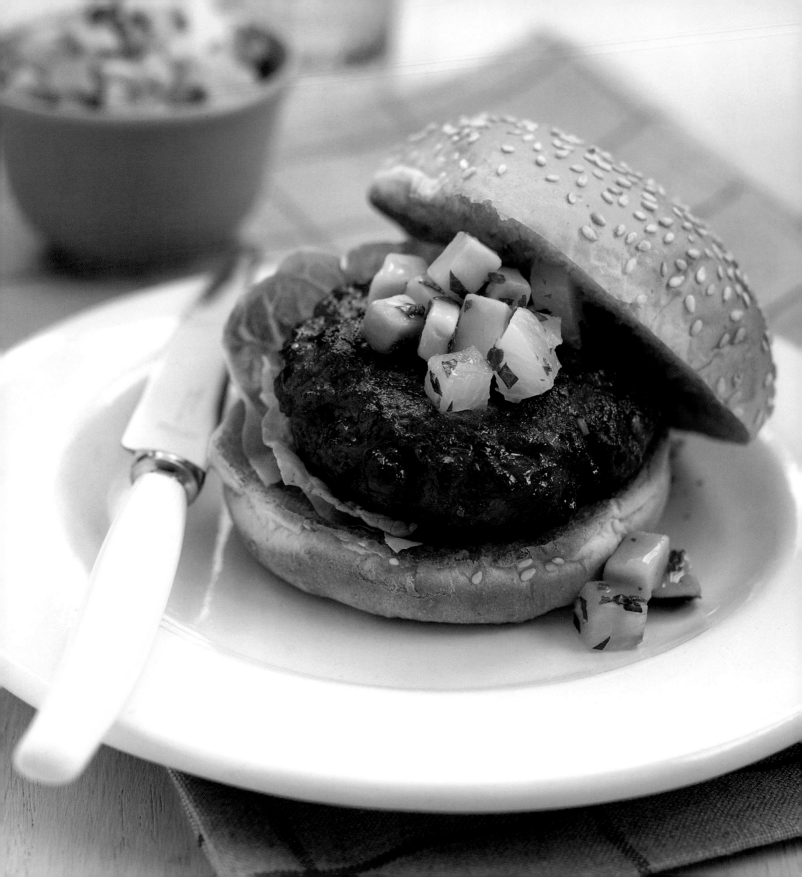

best burger with pineapple relish

1 lb lean ground beef, preferably hormone and antibiotic free

2 teaspoons chopped fresh oregano

1 large garlic clove, crushed (optional)

sea salt and freshly ground black pepper

PINEAPPLE RELISH

2½ oz. fresh pineapple, peeled, cored, and finely diced, or canned pineapple in natural juice

1 tablespoon chopped fresh mint

2 teaspoons freshly squeezed lemon juice

½ teaspoon dried hot pepper flakes (optional)

½ small avocado, pitted, peeled, and diced

TO SERVE

2 lettuce leaves

2 seeded or plain whole-wheat hamburger buns or rolls

SERVES 2

Longing for fast food? This burger will satisfy any craving, but without being detrimental to your health. It's made from good-lean ground beef and provides plenty of iron, a mineral found in a readily absorbable form in red meat. The tangy relish adds essential vitamins.

Mix together the ground beef, oregano, and garlic, if using, in a bowl. Season and divide the mixture in half. Use your hands to roll one half into a ball, then flatten into a burger shape and put it on a plate. Repeat to make one more burger. Cover with plastic wrap and chill in the fridge for 30 minutes.

Preheat the broiler to medium-high and line a broiler pan with foil. Meanwhile, mix together the ingredients for the relish and set aside to allow the flavors to merge.

Broil the burgers for 4–6 minutes each side until cooked through and there is no trace of pink in the center.

To serve, put a lettuce leaf on the bottom half of a hamburger bun. Put the burger on top and add a spoonful of the relish. Top with the second half of the bun. Serve with a side salad.

Red meat

Red meats such as beef, lamb, and pork can make a nutritious contribution to your diet during pregnancy. As well as protein, they are good providers of B vitamins and minerals such as zinc and readily absorbed iron. To help keep your saturated fat intake in check, trim meats well, and choose lean cuts and enjoy as part of a balanced meal.

mint and pea risotto

The peas and Parmesan in this vibrantly colored, classic Italian risotto provide a protein and mineral boost. The peas can be left whole, if preferred. Rice is a good source of energy-giving carbohydrate. Serve with a tomato salad to balance the meal.

1 tablespoon olive oil

1 large onion, finely chopped

1 cup arborio (risotto) rice

1⅔ cups frozen baby peas

¼ cup chopped fresh mint

a handful of fresh basil leaves, plus extra to garnish

3¾ cups hot vegetable broth

3 tablespoons finely grated Parmesan cheese, plus extra to serve

sea salt and freshly ground black pepper

SERVES 2

Heat the oil in a large heavy-based saucepan and sauté the onion, covered, for 12 minutes, stirring occasionally, until softened. Add the rice and stir for a couple of minutes until it is coated in the oil.

Meanwhile, steam the baby peas until tender, then transfer to a food processor with the mint, basil, and 3 tablespoons of the broth. Process until puréed, then set aside.

Add a ladleful of hot broth to the rice, then stir continuously with a wooden spoon until the rice has absorbed the liquid. Add the remaining broth, a ladleful at a time, stirring to allow the rice to cook evenly and to prevent it sticking to the bottom of the pan. Continue this process until all the broth is used and the rice is cooked and creamy but still retains a slight bite—this will take about 25 minutes.

Remove the pan from the heat and stir in the pea purée and the Parmesan. Season to taste and warm through gently. Serve sprinkled with extra Parmesan and basil leaves.

baked trout with ginger and orange dressing

Trout is part of the oily fish family and provides long-chain omega-3 fatty acids and valuable protein and minerals, while the noodles are a good source of carbohydrate. Serve with vitamin-rich steamed bok choy and broccoli, or a vegetable stir-fry.

sunflower or canola oil, for brushing

2 pink trout fillets, about 6 oz. each

6 oz. medium egg noodles

fresh cilantro leaves, to garnish

2 teaspoons toasted sesame seeds, to serve

sea salt and freshly ground black pepper

GINGER AND ORANGE DRESSING

1 tablespoon freshly squeezed lemon juice

2 tablespoons fresh orange juice (not from concentrate)

1 tablespoon honey

1 teaspoon sesame oil

1 tablespoon soy sauce

1 inch fresh ginger, peeled and cut into matchsticks

SERVES 2

Preheat the oven to 400°F. Lightly brush a baking pan with oil. Put the trout fillets in the pan, season, and bake for 10–12 minutes, depending on the thickness of the fillets, or until cooked.

Meanwhile, cook the noodles in plenty of boiling water following the instructions on the package until tender, then drain.

To make the dressing, put the lemon and orange juice, honey, sesame oil, soy sauce, and ginger in a small saucepan and bring to a boil. Reduce the heat and simmer, stirring occasionally, for about 3 minutes until reduced and slightly thickened.

Divide the noodles between 2 serving plates, top with the trout fillets, and spoon over the warm dressing. Sprinkle with the cilantro and sesame seeds before serving.

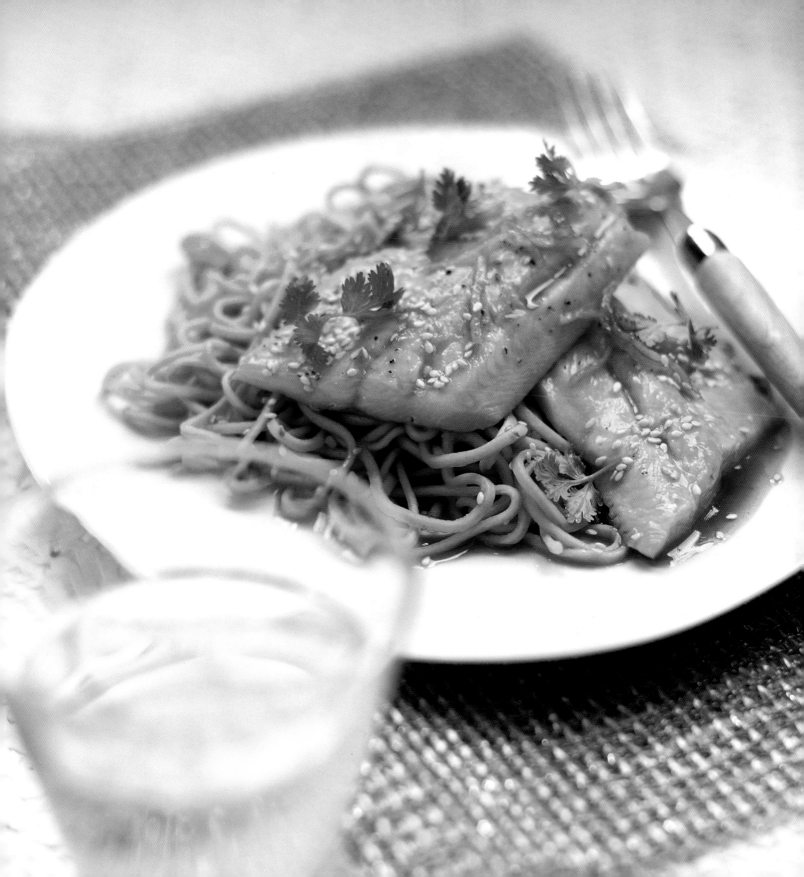

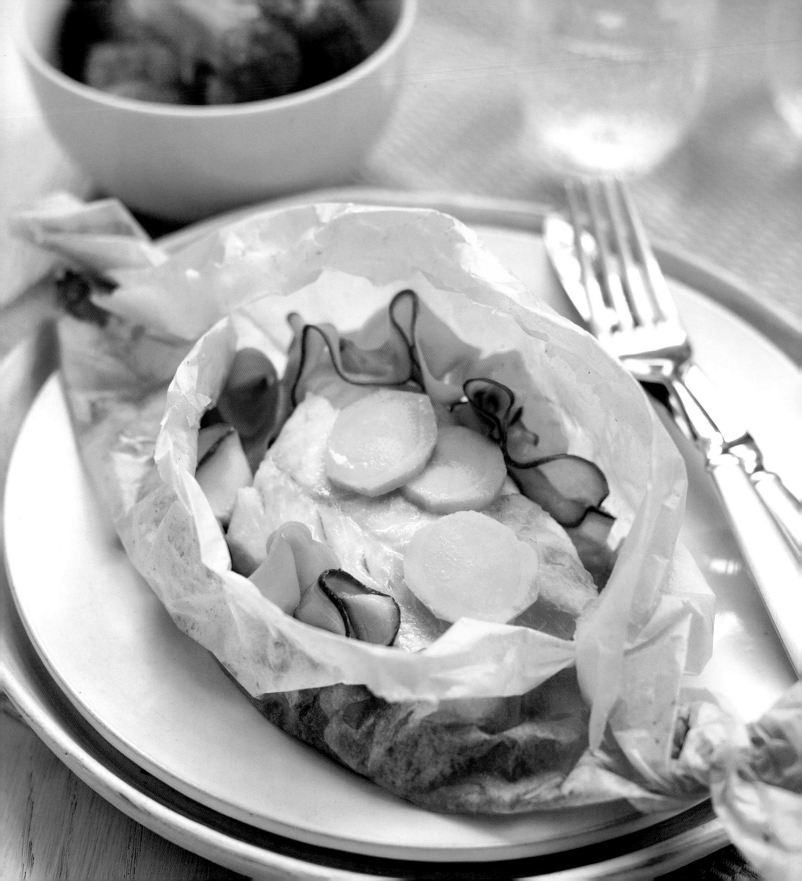

sesame ginger fish

Delicately flavored, this is a perfect light and healthy supper, especially if you are feeling off or have indigestion. For a balanced meal, serve with new potatoes, noodles, or rice, and steamed broccoli.

1 tablespoon soy sauce

1½ teaspoons toasted sesame oil

1 zucchini, cut into ribbons

1 carrot, peeled and cut into ribbons

2 tilapia or other firm white fish fillets, about 6 oz. each

6 x ½ inch slices peeled fresh ginger

sea salt and freshly ground black pepper

SERVES 2

Mix together the soy sauce and sesame oil.

Put half of the zucchini and carrot ribbons in the center of a sheet of parchment paper that is large enough to make a package. Put a tilapia fillet on top of the vegetables, then 3 slices of ginger. Repeat with the remaining ingredients to make a second package.

Spoon the soy sauce mixture over the fish. Gather up the paper around the fish and fold over to seal and make 2 loose packages.

Put the fish packages in a steamer, cover, and steam for 10–15 minutes, depending on the thickness of the fillets, until cooked. Open up the packages, then season to taste before serving.

roast chicken
with tomato pesto

The sun-dried tomato pesto topping keeps the chicken deliciously moist during roasting, as well as providing a beneficial cocktail of antioxidants and minerals. The pesto can also be mixed into pasta or spooned on top of a baked potato. It will keep for up to a week in an airtight container in the fridge.

2 skinless, boneless chicken breasts, about 6 oz. each

5 oz. fresh spinach, Swiss chard, or Savoy cabbage, shredded

a squeeze of fresh lemon juice

fresh basil leaves, to garnish

1 tablespoon toasted pine nuts, to serve

TOMATO PESTO

2 oz. sun-dried tomatoes in oil

1 garlic clove, crushed

2 tablespoons pine nuts

1 tablespoon extra virgin olive oil

sea salt and freshly ground black pepper

SERVES 2

Preheat the oven to 400°F.

To make the tomato pesto, drain the sun-dried tomatoes and reserve 1 tablespoon of the oil. Put the sun-dried tomatoes in a food processor with the reserved oil, garlic, pine nuts, olive oil, and 1 tablespoon water. Process until you have a coarse paste, then season to taste.

Put the chicken in a lightly oiled roasting pan. Spread the tomato pesto over the top of each chicken breast. Cover the pan with foil.

Roast the chicken for 10 minutes, then remove the foil. Return the chicken to the oven and cook for another 10–15 minutes until cooked through and there is no sign of pink in the center.

Meanwhile, steam the spinach until tender and squeeze over a little lemon juice. Divide between 2 plates and top with the chicken breasts. Drizzle over any juices left in the tray and sprinkle with the basil leaves and pine nuts before serving.

lemon and spinach Puy lentils with egg

Puy lentils have a slightly firm texture and nutty flavor, and retain their shape when cooked. Like other types of lentil, they are a low-fat, nutritious source of fiber, protein, folic acid, and iron. Eggs are a good source of choline, which is believed to help with brain development in the growing foetus.

¾ cup Puy or other green lentils, rinsed

1 large bay leaf

1 tablespoon olive oil

1 large onion, roughly chopped

5 vine-ripened tomatoes, halved, seeded, and cut into chunks

5 oz. fresh spinach, thinly sliced

2 heaping teaspoons Dijon mustard

2 tablespoons reduced-fat crème fraîche

freshly squeezed juice of 1 lemon

sea salt and freshly ground black pepper

2–3 large hard-cooked free-range eggs, to serve

SERVES 2–3

Put the lentils and bay leaf in a saucepan. Cover with cold water and bring to a boil. Reduce the heat, half-cover the pan, and cook for 25–30 minutes until tender but not mushy. Drain the lentils and set aside.

Meanwhile, heat the oil in a sauté pan and fry the onion, covered, for 10 minutes until softened. Add the tomatoes and spinach to the pan and cook, stirring, for another 2 minutes until the spinach has wilted.

Add the cooked lentils to the pan with the Dijon mustard, crème fraîche, and lemon juice, stirring until everything is combined. Season to taste and warm through.

Spoon the lentils onto 2 or 3 serving plates. Halve the hard-cooked eggs and place on top of the lentils before serving.

grilled pork with mashed sweet potatoes

Pure comfort food! Orange-fleshed sweet potatoes contain many antioxidants, including vitamin C. Serve the pork with your favorite green vegetable.

1½ tablespoons olive oil, plus extra if needed

½ teaspoon paprika

2 pork loin fillets, 5 oz. each

sea salt and freshly ground black pepper

SERVES 2

SWEET POTATO MASH

1 lb. orange-fleshed sweet potatoes, peeled and cut into chunks

2 teaspoons butter

4 tablespoons chopped fresh cilantro, plus extra sprigs to garnish

a ridged stovetop grill pan

Mix together 1 tablespoon of the oil and the paprika and brush the mixture over the pork. Season to taste.

Cook the sweet potatoes in boiling salted water until tender. Drain, then return the potatoes to the pan. Add the butter and remaining oil and mash the potatoes until smooth and creamy. Stir in the chopped cilantro and season to taste.

Meanwhile, heat a stovetop grill pan until very hot. Grill the pork for 5–6 minutes or until cooked right through, turning halfway and brushing with more oil, if necessary.

Divide the mashed sweet potatoes between 2 plates, then top with the pork and garnish with extra cilantro sprigs.

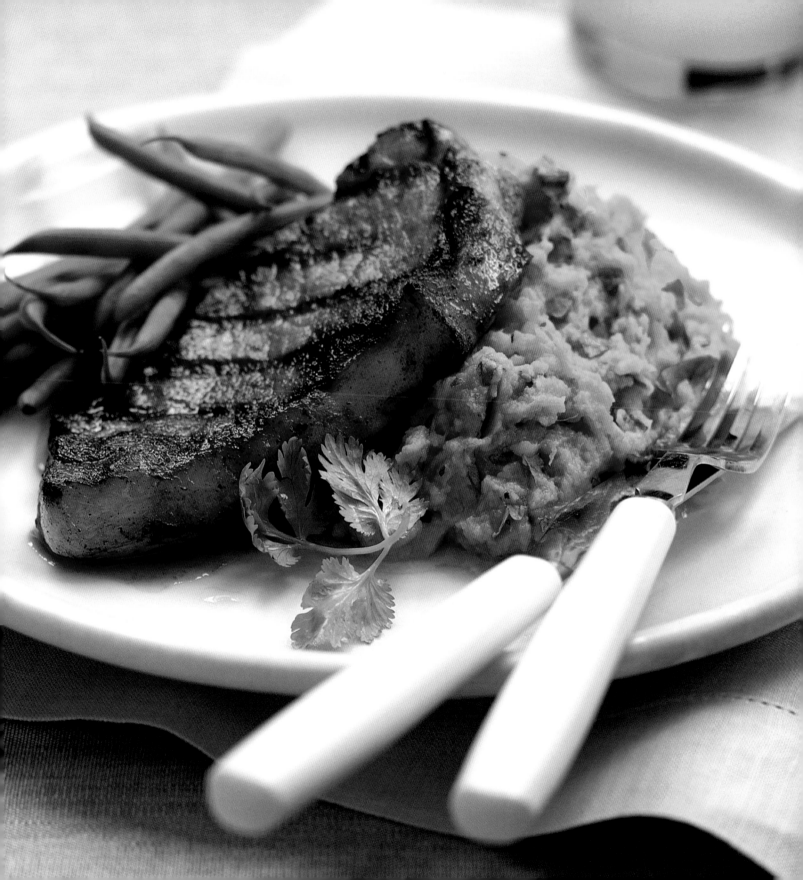

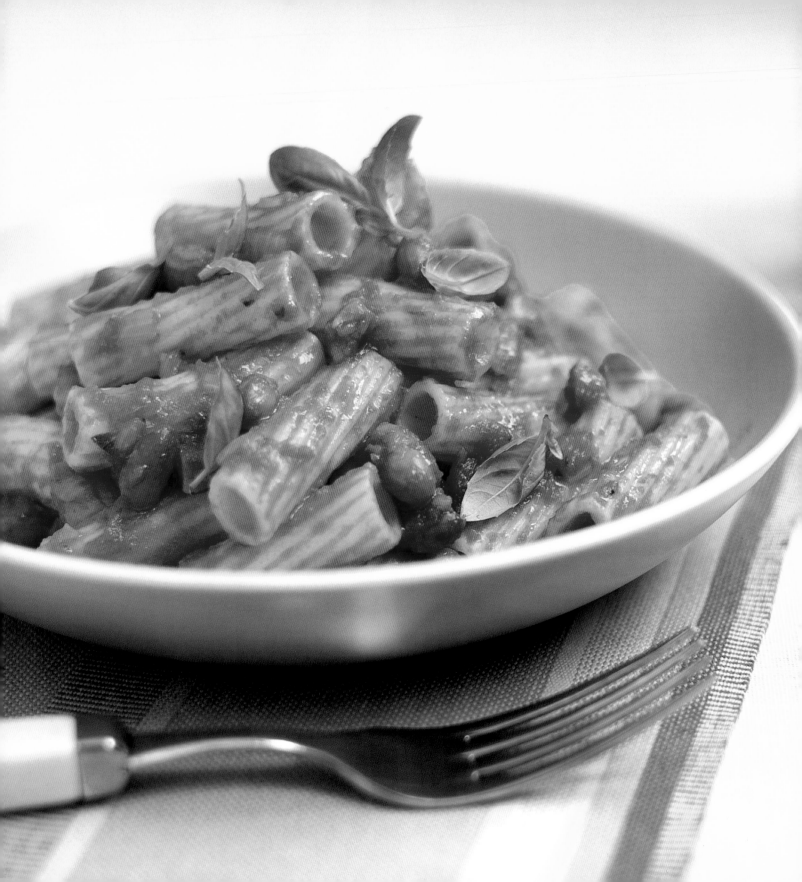

rigatoni with pancetta and beans

1 tablespoon olive oil

1 onion, chopped

1 garlic clove, finely chopped

1 teaspoon dried oregano

4½ oz. pancetta or lean smoky bacon, roughly chopped

1⅔ cups passata

a pinch of sugar

1 teaspoon tomato paste

3½ oz. canned borlotti beans, drained and rinsed

6½ oz. dried rigatoni

sea salt and freshly ground black pepper

SERVES 2

Rustic and hearty, this pasta dish makes a warming dinner. Canned beans are a convenient pantry standby, and as well as providing slow release energy and low-fat protein, three heaped tablespoons count as a single portion of the recommended "five-a-day."

Heat the oil in a saucepan and fry the onion for 8 minutes until softened, then stir in the garlic, oregano, and pancetta and cook for another 2 minutes.

Pour in the passata and stir in the sugar and tomato paste. Bring to a boil, then reduce the heat to low and simmer, half-covered, for 10 minutes, stirring occasionally. Add the beans, stir and cook for another 5 minutes.

Meanwhile, cook the pasta in plenty of boiling salted water, following the instructions on the package, until al dente. Drain, reserving ¼ cup of the cooking water. Set aside.

Add the cooked pasta and reserved cooking water to the sauce and heat through before serving. Season to taste.

Legumes

Legumes are the edible seeds of pod-bearing plants such as peas, beans, chickpeas, and lentils. Peanuts are also a type of legume. Nutritionally, they are an alternative to lean meat or fish. This means they are great for protein, along with B vitamins (except for B_{12}), and minerals such as iron and zinc. They also have the added benefit of packing in antioxidants, fiber, and slow release carbohydrates. Enjoy them in meat-free meals or use alongside smaller amounts of meat in a recipe.

grilled mackerel with citrus salsa

4 mackerel fillets, boned, about
6 oz. each

sea salt and freshly ground
black pepper

olive oil, for brushing

CITRUS SALSA

2 oranges, peeled, segmented,
and diced

1 shallot, finely diced (optional)

½ mild red chile, seeded and
diced (optional)

freshly squeezed juice and zest
of 1 lime

1 tablespoon olive oil

3 tablespoons chopped fresh mint

SERVES 2

Compared to other types of oily fish (*see* page 29), mackerel is one of the richest sources of long-chain omega-3 fatty acids. The zingy citrus salsa complements the richness of this economical fish and adds valuable vitamin C. Serve with whole-grain bread and a green salad.

Preheat the broiler to high and line a broiler pan with foil.

Meanwhile, make the salsa. Put the oranges, shallot, chile, if using, lime juice and zest, oil, and mint into a non-metallic bowl. Stir until the ingredients are combined. Set aside to allow the flavors to mingle.

Brush the mackerel with oil and season, then broil for about 2 minutes each side. Serve with spoonfuls of the citrus salsa.

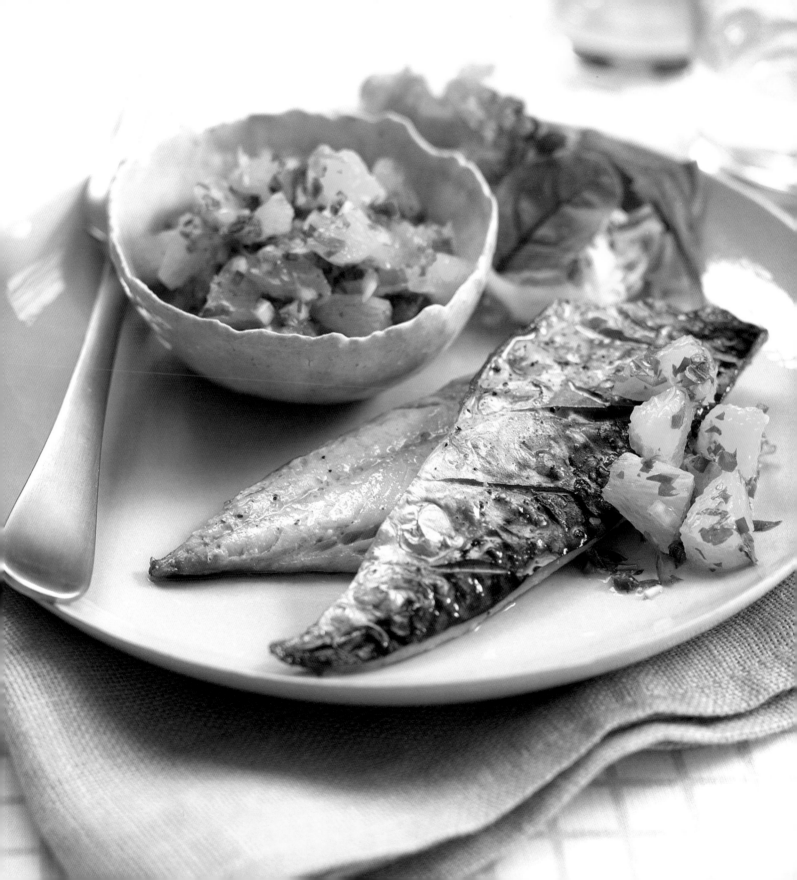

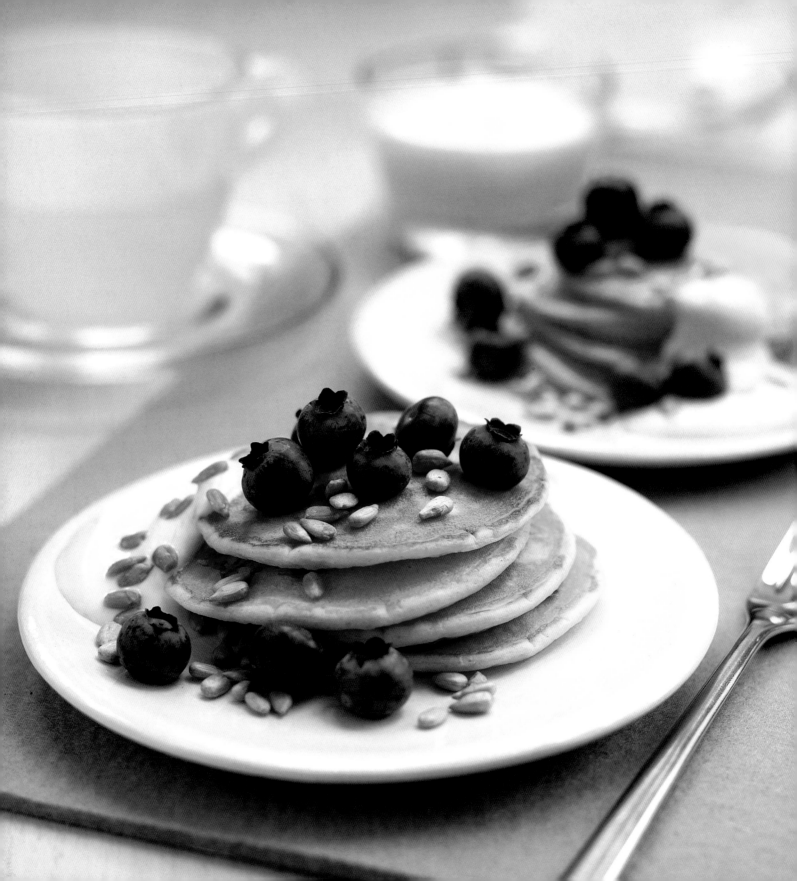

sweet things

pancakes with blueberries

Pancakes aren't just for breakfast! Serve warm with a sprinkling of sunflower seeds and blueberries to boost your antioxidant intake (vitamins C and E). A spoonful of yogurt adds the finishing touch.

1 cup plus 1 tablespoon self-rising flour

2 tablespoons sugar

a pinch of salt

⅔ cup low-fat milk

1 large free-range egg, lightly beaten

4 heaping tablespoons thick, plain low-fat yogurt, plus extra to serve

sunflower or canola oil, for frying

fresh blueberries and toasted sunflower seeds, to serve

MAKES 10 PANCAKES

SERVES 3

Sift the flour into a large mixing bowl. Stir in the sugar and salt and make a well in the center of the mixture.

Pour the milk into a glass measuring cup and beat in the egg. Gradually pour the egg mixture into the mixing bowl, stirring continuously until you have a smooth batter. Stir in the yogurt, then allow the batter to rest for 30 minutes.

Heat a little oil in a large nonstick skillet. Spoon a small ladleful of batter into the skillet to make a pancake about 2½ inches in diameter. Cook 3 pancakes at a time for about 1½ minutes each side until golden. Keep them warm while you make the remaining pancakes.

Serve 3–4 pancakes per person, accompanied by the blueberries, a spoonful of yogurt, and a sprinkling of toasted sunflower seeds.

carrot and walnut muffins

9 tablespoons unsalted butter or polyunsaturated margarine

2½ cups all-purpose flour (or half and half all-purpose and whole-wheat flour)

1½ teaspoons apple pie spice

1 tablespoon baking powder

¾ cup light brown sugar

8 oz. carrots, peeled and grated

⅓ cup walnuts, chopped (optional)

2 large free-range eggs, lightly beaten

5–6 tablespoons low-fat milk

12 walnut halves, to decorate

TOPPING

¼ cup low-fat cream cheese

2 tablespoons butter or polyunsaturated margarine

3 tablespoons confectioners' sugar

½ teaspoon pure vanilla extract

MAKES 12

a deep, 12-holed muffin pan, lined with paper cases

a wire rack

Light yet satisfyingly indulgent, the carrots in these muffins provide the valuable antioxidant beta-carotene, which as a general rule is more readily absorbed from cooked foods, and later converted to vitamin A in the body. Walnuts are one of the few nuts to contain useful amounts of omega-3 fatty acids. Try not to over-mix the muffin mixture, as this can give them a heavy texture.

Preheat the oven to 400°F.

Melt the butter in a small saucepan over gentle heat, then let cool slightly.

Meanwhile, sift the flour, apple pie spice, and baking powder into a large mixing bowl. Stir in the brown sugar, carrots, and chopped walnuts, if using.

Pour the butter into the flour mixture with the eggs and milk and mix gently with a wooden spoon until combined.

Spoon the mixture into the paper cases, then bake for 20 minutes until risen and golden. Transfer to a wire rack to cool.

To make the topping, beat together the cream cheese, butter, confectioners' sugar, and pure vanilla extract until smooth and creamy. Spread the cream cheese mixture on top of the muffins, then decorate each with a walnut half.

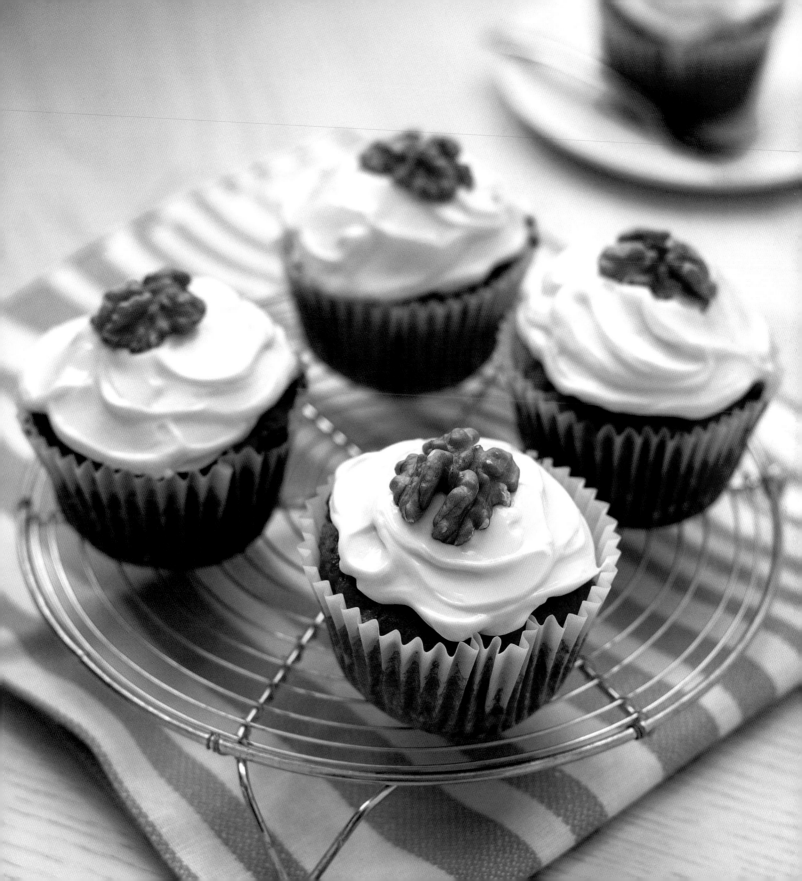

strawberry sundae

Layers of fresh strawberry sauce and crushed amaretti biscuits are interspersed with creamy vanilla yogurt custard to make a delicious dessert with plenty of nutritional attributes.

2¼ cups strawberries, hulled

8 oz. (1 cup) vanilla yogurt

¾ cup low-fat Greek yogurt

½ teaspoon pure vanilla extract (optional)

6 amaretti biscuits, roughly broken

SERVES 2

2 sundae glasses

Set aside 4 strawberries to decorate. Purée the remaining fruit in a blender or by pressing it through a sieve. (If using a blender or food processor, you may wish to press the strawberry purée through a sieve to remove any seeds.) Set aside.

Mix together the vanilla yogurt, Greek yogurt, and pure vanilla extract, if using, in a bowl.

Spoon a layer of the yogurt mixture into two tall glasses. Top with a layer of strawberry purée and amaretti biscuits. Repeat with another layer of yogurt mixture, the remaining purée, and amaretti. Top with a final layer of yogurt mixture.

Slice the reserved strawberries and use to decorate the sundaes.

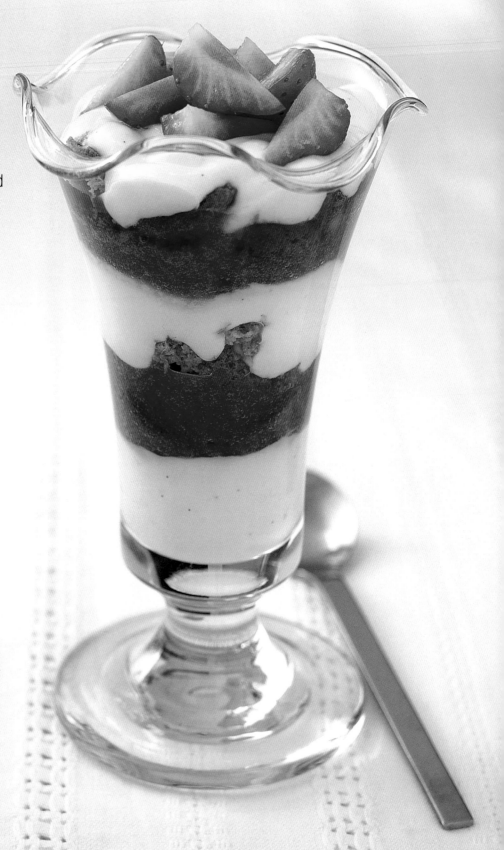

cinnamon French toast with bananas

1 large free-range egg, lightly beaten

¼ cup low-fat milk

2 teaspoons butter or
polyunsaturated margarine

2 cinnamon raisin English muffins,
halved horizontally

TO SERVE

1 large banana, diagonally sliced

2 teaspoons pure maple syrup

¼ cup low-fat Greek yogurt

2 large pinches of ground cinnamon

SERVES 2

The bananas and fromage frais in this tasty twist on French toast provide an added nutrition boost. This dish can also be enjoyed as a lazy Sunday morning brunch.

Use a fork to mix together the egg and milk in a shallow dish. Melt the butter in a large nonstick skillet and swirl it around to coat the base evenly.

Dip both sides of the muffin halves in the egg mixture, then allow any excess to drip off.

Put the muffins in the skillet and cook each side for about 2 minutes, or until the egg has set and they are light golden.

Put 2 muffin halves on each serving plate and top with the banana slices, then drizzle over the maple syrup. Serve with the Greek yogurt and sprinkle with the ground cinnamon.

stem ginger and apricot cookies

6½ tablespoons unsalted butter or polyunsaturated margarine

6 tablespoons light brown sugar

⅔ cup self-rising flour

3 tablespoons whole-wheat self-rising flour

⅔ cup old-fashioned rolled oats

2 oz. stem ginger, roughly chopped

2½ oz. ready-to-eat unsulfured dried apricots, roughly chopped

MAKES 16

2 baking sheets, lined with parchment paper

a wire rack

If you're suffering from morning sickness, a cookie or biscuit may help settle the stomach. These contain stem ginger, which is known for its anti-nausea properties.

Preheat the oven to 350°F.

Cream the butter and sugar together in a bowl using a wooden spoon or hand-held mixer until light and fluffy. Sift in both types of flour, then gently stir in with the oats, stem ginger, and dried apricots to make a softish dough.

Put tablespoons of the cookie mixture onto the lined baking sheets, making sure they are well spaced out to allow room for them to spread. Slightly flatten the top of each cookie, then bake for 15–20 minutes until light golden but still slightly soft.

Let cool for 5 minutes, then transfer to a wire rack to cool completely.

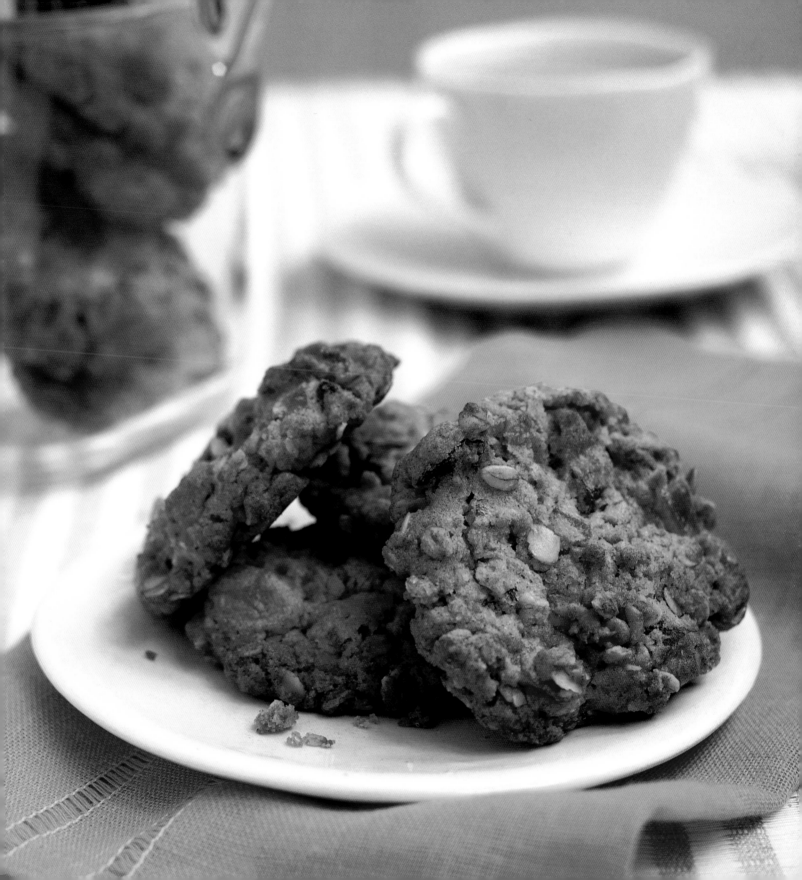

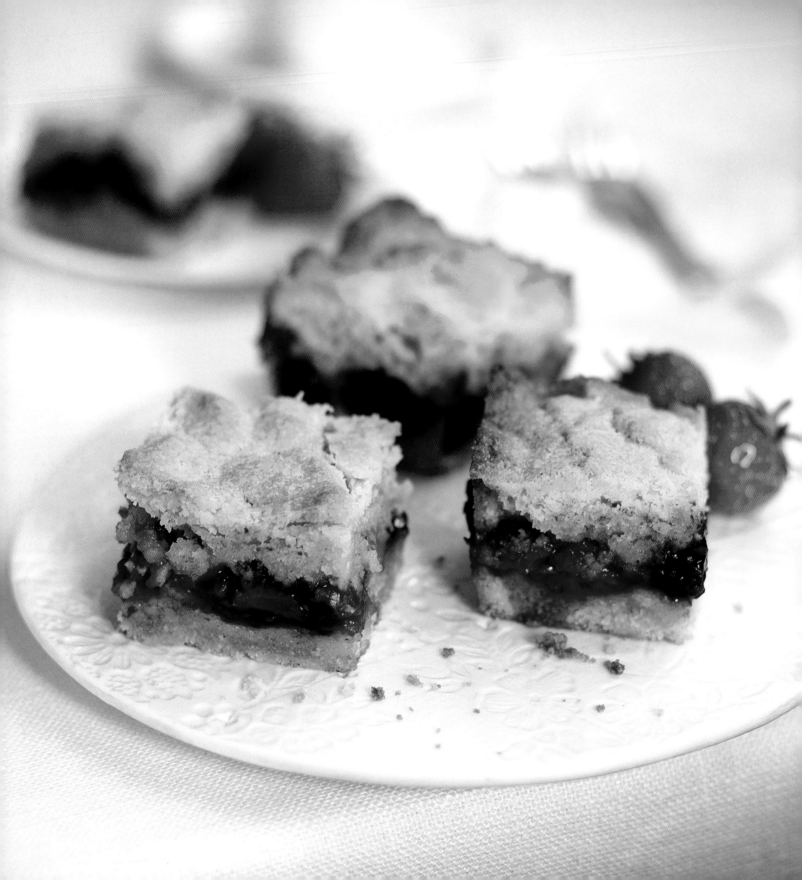

summer fruit bars

These bars have a fruity surprise sandwiched in the center—a juicy layer of summer berries. Serve them with an extra helping of vitamin C-rich berries. A scoop of vanilla ice cream is also delicious. If fresh berries are out of season, you can use frozen fruit instead (bags of frozen mixed berries are nutritious and very convenient).

2 cups all-purpose flour

1⅓ cups ground almonds

2 sticks unsalted butter or polyunsaturated margarine

1 cup sugar

2 free-range eggs

10 oz. mixed summer berries, such as raspberries, strawberries, and blackberries, plus extra to serve

MAKES 16 BARS

an 8 inch square cake pan, buttered and base-lined with baking parchment

a wire rack

Preheat the oven to 350°F.

Put the flour, almonds, butter, sugar, and eggs in a food processor and mix to a soft dough. Divide the mixture in half.

Press one half of the dough into the prepared pan. The easiest way to do this is to take a small handful of dough, flatten it slightly in your hand, then press it into the pan. Repeat to make an even layer about ½ inch thick. Lightly press the summer berries into the dough in an even layer. Top the fruit with the remaining dough, covering it in an even layer using the method above.

Put the pan in the center of the oven and bake for 35–40 minutes until the top is light golden. Remove from the oven and transfer to a wire rack to cool for 10 minutes.

To remove the cake from the pan, put the wire rack on top of the pan and carefully turn it over so the rack is on the bottom—the cake should pop out of the pan. Peel away the parchment lining, then turn the cake over. Cut into 16 squares and serve with berries.

Sweet as sugar

Sugar is a type of carbohydrate and comes in many different forms. Fructose, for example, is naturally found in fruit and honey, and lactose is naturally present in milk. Sucrose is table sugar and, like other forms of sugar (e.g. dextrose, glucose syrup), is added to confectionery, baked goods, and processed foods and drinks. Modest amounts of added sugar (up to 12 teaspoons daily) in a balanced diet are fine, but many of us overdo it. It's wise to keep a limit on sugary snacks and drinks. Consuming them frequently can promote tooth decay, and they may also be high in fat and calories and low in nutrients. If you do fancy something sweet at the end of a meal, a portion of one of the desserts from this book will not only satisfy your sweet tooth, but will also provide nutrition.

grilled peaches with pistachios and dates

2 heaping tablespoons low-fat cream cheese

2 teaspoons fresh orange juice (not from concentrate)

10 pistachio nuts or other favorite nuts, roughly chopped

2 pitted dates, finely chopped

2 ripe peaches or nectarines

SERVES 2

A delicious, easy dessert of peaches stuffed with a creamy, nutritious date and nut filling. The perfect treat for those who don't want to spend long in the kitchen.

Preheat the broiler to medium and line a broiler pan with foil.

Meanwhile, mix together the cream cheese, orange juice, pistachios, and dates in a small bowl.

Cut the peaches in half lengthwise, twist to separate the fruit into halves, then pry out the pit.

Spoon the cream cheese mixture into the peach centers. Broil for 6–7 minutes until the cream cheese mixture starts to turn golden and the fruit softens.

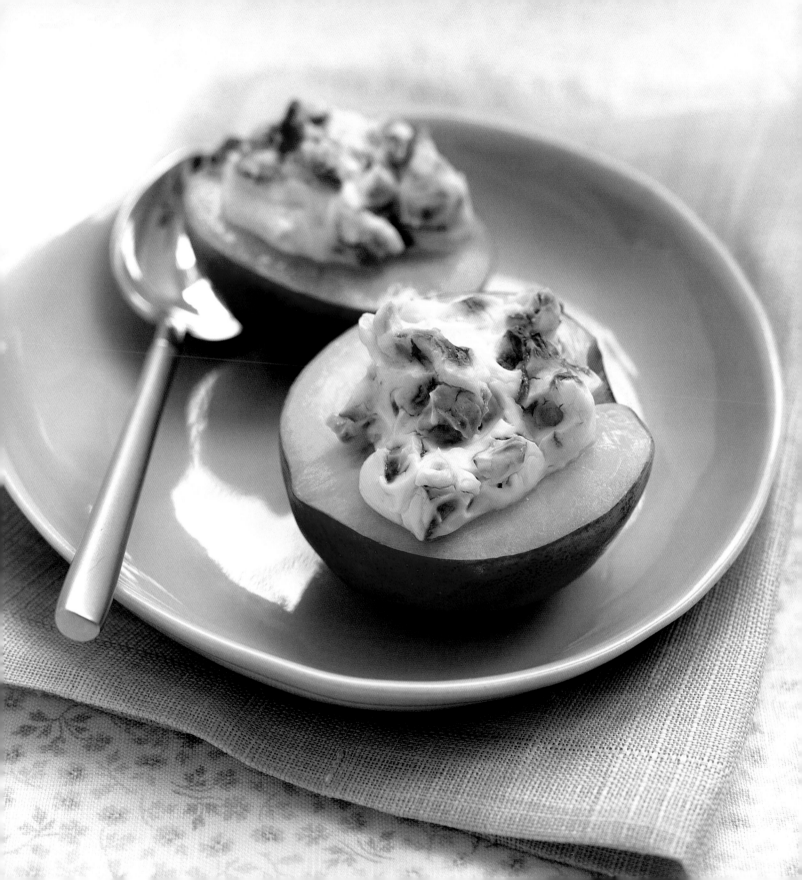

mango and honey yogurt ice

This refreshing, cooling yogurt ice comes with an antioxidant-rich mango sauce, although it tastes just as good served on its own. Likewise, the mango sauce can be served spooned over low-fat Greek yogurt. The yogurt ice also makes a nutritious snack, and an ideal standby for those slightly queasy days.

1 large ripe mango, pitted, peeled, and cubed (*see page 139*)

2 bananas, cut into chunks

2 cups thick, vanilla low-fat yogurt

3–4 tablespoons honey, to taste

a squeeze of fresh lemon juice

SIMPLE MANGO SAUCE

1 ripe mango, pitted, peeled, and sliced (optional)

SERVES 6–8

an ice cream maker (optional)

Put the mango and bananas in a food processor with the yogurt, honey, and lemon juice. Process until the fruit is puréed and the mixture is thick and creamy. Taste for sweetness—it should taste sweet—and add a little more honey if necessary.

Pour the mixture into an ice cream maker and churn following the manufacturer's instructions. Alternatively, pour it into a shallow, lidded freezerproof container and freeze. Beat or stir briskly with a fork every 2 hours to break up any ice crystals that have formed until the yogurt ice is frozen—this will help to give it a creamy texture.

Remove the yogurt ice from the freezer 30 minutes before eating to allow it to soften.

To make the mango sauce, if using, purée the mango in a food processor until smooth. Serve the yogurt ice in scoops with the mango sauce spooned over the top.

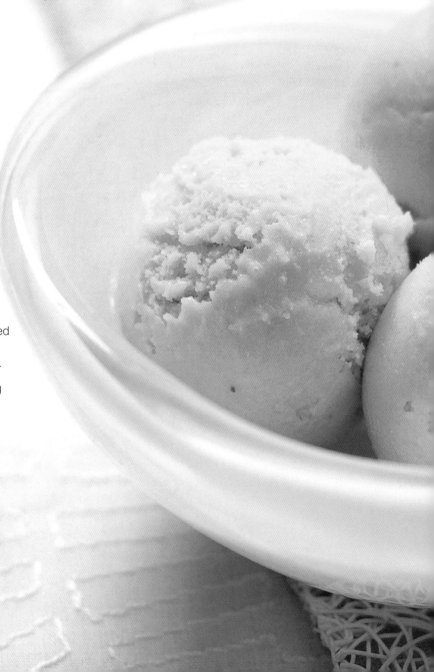

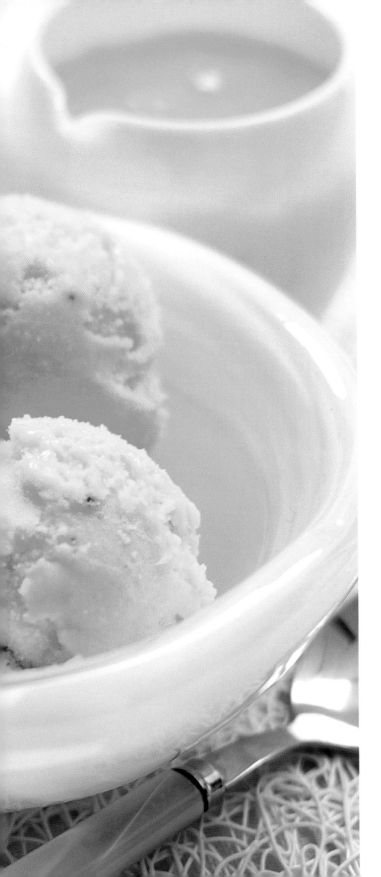

energy bars

One of these oat, apple, and seed bars is just the thing for an energy-sustaining, between-meal snack, and would also make a quick breakfast, served with a fruit smoothie or yogurt.

6½ tablespoons unsalted butter or polyunsaturated margarine

½ cup light brown sugar

¼ cup golden syrup or corn syrup

2 cups old-fashioned rolled oats

1 tablespoon hemp seeds or flaxseed

1 tablespoon pumpkin seeds

2 tablespoons sunflower seeds

1 apple, cored and grated

MAKES 16 BARS

an 8-inch square cake pan, buttered and base-lined with baking parchment

Preheat the oven to 350°F.

Meanwhile, melt the butter in a saucepan over gentle heat and add the sugar and syrup. Heat until just warm, stirring, until the sugar and syrup have melted.

Put the oats, seeds, and apple in a mixing bowl and pour the buttery mixture into the bowl. Mix with a wooden spoon until everything is combined, then spoon the mixture into the prepared pan.

Bake for 25–30 minutes until golden and slightly crisp. Slice into 16 bars while still warm and leave in the pan until cool and crisp.

Fats of life

We all need some fat in our diet to absorb fat-soluble vitamins, build cell membranes, and provide essential fatty acids that the body can't make. We also need some fat stores to insulate and cushion the body, and make vital hormones. The trick is not to overdo it (a high-fat diet promotes excess weight gain) and to opt for healthier fats. Different fats affect our health in different ways. Too many saturated fats or trans fats, found in fatty meats, pastries, crackers, cream, and full-fat dairy foods, can raise cholesterol levels. But switching to beneficial unsaturated fats, found in olive and canola oil, polyunsaturated spreads, oily fish, nuts, seeds, and avocados, can help heart health and provide essential fatty acids. Omega-3 fatty acids (*see* page 17) have a number of benefits for you and your developing baby.

rhubarb, pear, and ginger crumble

These individual fruity desserts contain the healthy addition of oats and sunflower seeds in the crumble topping. If rhubarb is not in season, plums, apples, and blackberries are equally delicious. The crumbles can be frozen, uncooked, for up to three months.

Preheat the oven to 400°F.

Put the rhubarb, pears, orange juice, sugar, and ginger in a large bowl and stir until everything is combined. Pack the fruit and any juice into the heatproof dishes until the fruit nearly reaches the top.

To make the crumble, put the flour, oats, seeds, sugar, and butter in a mixing bowl and rub them together with your fingertips until they form a coarse, chunky bread crumb texture—you don't want the crumble topping to be too fine in texture. (This can also be done in a food processor.)

Sprinkle the crumble mixture over the fruit. Put the dishes on a baking sheet and bake the crumbles for 25–30 minutes until the tops are golden.

6 oz. rhubarb, sliced into bite-size pieces

2 pears, peeled, cored, and cut into bite-size pieces

5 tablespoons fresh orange juice (not from concentrate)

1 tablespoon light brown sugar

1 teaspoon ground ginger

CRUMBLE TOPPING

¾ cup all-purpose flour

⅓ cup old-fashioned rolled oats

1 tablespoon sunflower seeds

6 tablespoons coarse raw sugar

4 tablespoons cold unsalted butter, cubed

SERVES 4

4 x 6-oz. heatproof dishes

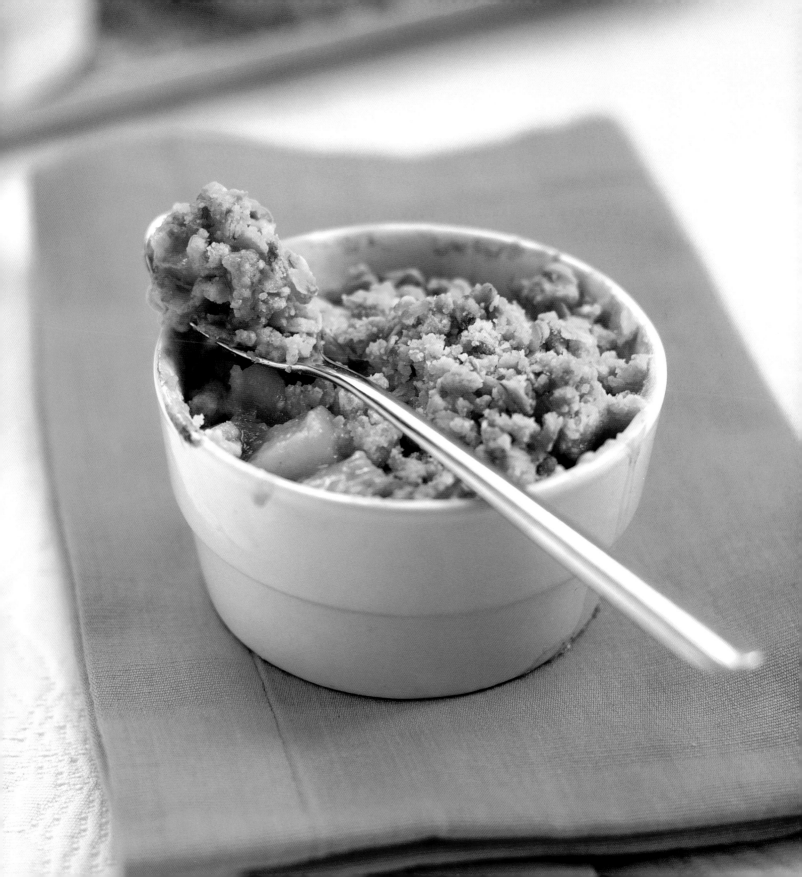

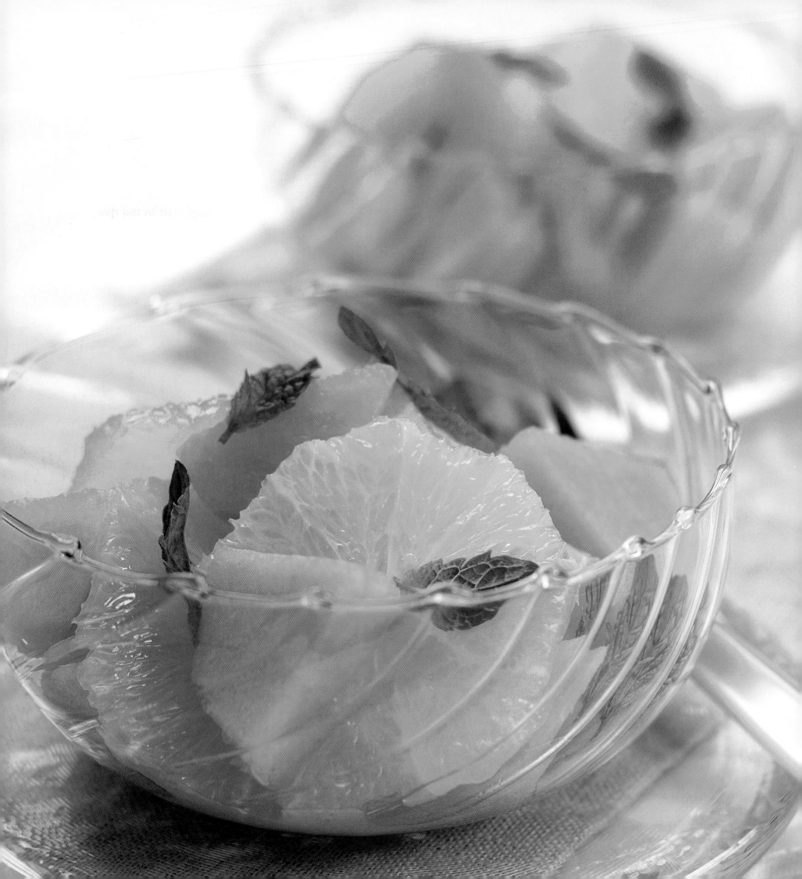

citrus and melon fruit salad with mint

Refreshing and packed with beta-carotene (an antioxidant that the body can also convert to vitamin A) and vitamin C, this recipe is great for the skin and immune system. A sprinkling of fresh mint, a traditional digestive, complements the fruit salad.

1 orange

1 wedge cantaloupe

6 fresh mint leaves, torn

SERVES 1

Slice off the orange peel and any remaining pith. Thinly slice the orange into rounds. Put the orange slices and any juice in a shallow bowl.

Remove the skin from the melon and cut into bite-size chunks. Add to the orange and sprinkle the mint over the top. Best served right away.

Vitamin C, beta-carotene, lycopene

Sweet and juicy, cantaloupe melon is bursting with vitamin C and beta-carotene, which accounts for its distinctive orange flesh. Red watermelon contains the powerful antioxidant lycopene, also abundant in rosy red tomatoes. Melon is wonderfully soothing too, and a fruit that many find easiest to manage if feeling a bit nauseous. As well as adding zest and color to a fruit salad, keep cut-up cubes in a sealed container in the fridge, or add to a fruit smoothie.

fruit and nut bars

Packed with energy-giving and iron-boosting dried fruit and fabulously nutritious nuts and seeds, one of these simple-to-prepare bars would make an excellent snack, or pair one with a smoothie or some yogurt for a convenient start to the day.

3 tablespoons hazelnuts, roughly chopped

3 tablespoons Brazil nuts, roughly chopped

⅓ cup old-fashioned rolled oats

½ cup raisins

¾ cup unsulfured dried apricots,
cut into small pieces

¼ cup fresh orange juice (not from concentrate)

2 tablespoons sunflower seeds

2 tablespoons pumpkin seeds

MAKES 8 BARS

7 x 10 inch baking pan, lined with rice paper

Put the nuts and oats in a dry skillet and toast over medium heat for 3 minutes, turning them occasionally with a wooden spatula until they begin to turn golden and the oats become crisp. Remove from the skillet and let cool.

Put the raisins, apricots, and orange juice in a food processor and purée until the mixture becomes a smooth, thick purée. Scrape the fruit purée into a mixing bowl.

Put the nuts, oats, and seeds in the food processor and process until they are very finely chopped. Tip the mixture into the bowl with the fruit purée. Stir until all the ingredients are combined.

Tip the fruit and nut mixture into the prepared pan and, using a palette knife, smooth in an even layer about ½ inch thick. Chill in the fridge for 1 hour before cutting into 8 bars.

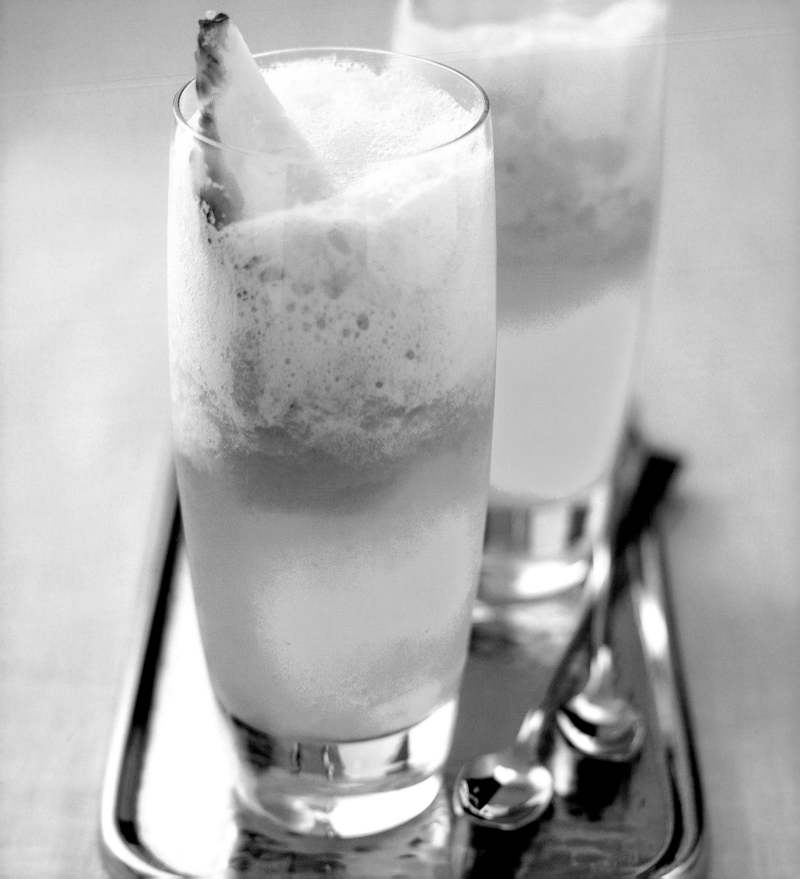

drinks

pineapple and ginger crush

It can be difficult to find long, refreshing, non-alcoholic drinks, but this tempting fruit crush will satisfy your thirst. The ginger may help settle any nausea.

2 cups fresh pineapple, peeled, cored, and cubed

2 teaspoons grated fresh ginger

chilled ginger ale

2 wedges of fresh pineapple, to serve

SERVES 2

Finely chop the pineapple cubes in a food processor. Combine with the ginger, then spoon the mixture into a small freezer proof container with a lid. Freeze for 2 hours until the mixture forms ice crystals.

Remove from the freezer and mix with a fork to break up the ice crystals, then divide the mixture between 2 tall glasses. Top up with ginger ale and serve with a wedge of pineapple.

lemon and ginger infusion

Excellent first thing or mid-morning, this refreshing drink is ideal if you're feeling nauseous or a little groggy.

1 inch fresh ginger, peeled and cut into thin rounds

1 cup just-boiled water

1 tablespoon freshly squeezed lemon juice

2 slices of lemon

SERVES 1

Put the ginger in a mug or small teapot and pour over the hot water. Put the lid on the teapot, if using, and let steep for 10 minutes.

Remove all but 2 slices of the ginger, if making it in a mug, or pour the liquid into a cup and add a couple of the ginger slices. Add the lemon juice and slices of lemon.

chamomile and lemon balm infusion

Perfect before bed, lemon balm and chamomile have long been known for their calming qualities, and may help to aid restful sleep.

1 lemon balm tea bag

1 chamomile tea bag

1 cup just-boiled water

1 slice of lemon

SERVES 1

Put the lemon balm and chamomile tea bags into a mug or small teapot and pour over the hot water. Put the lid on the teapot, if using, and let steep for 10 minutes.

Remove the bags from the mug, or pour the tea into a cup, and add a slice of lemon.

Herbal teas

Always check unusual herbal teas or preparations with your herbalist, midwife, or pharmacist. Some herbal preparations, such as black cohosh and feverfew, should be totally avoided during pregnancy. Caffeine-free herbal tea bags are an alternative to tea and coffee. As a general rule, everyday herbal tea bags you buy from supermarkets are fine, such as chamomile or peppermint, as is ginger "tea" made with a little fresh ginger. But since all herbs contain bioactive compounds, it is still best to keep to moderate daily amounts.

peppermint and ginger infusion

Caffeine-free herb infusions are an alternative to tea and coffee and can have beneficial qualities. This tea combines peppermint and ginger—both may help to calm nausea, while peppermint may ease bloating (but note that it could make heartburn worse).

Put the peppermint tea bag into a mug or small teapot. Pour over the hot water. Add the ginger and put the lid on the teapot, if using. Steep for 10 minutes.

Remove the tea bag and all but 2 slices of the ginger from the mug, or pour the tea from the teapot into a cup and add a couple of the ginger slices.

1 peppermint tea bag

1 cup just-boiled water

1 inch fresh ginger, peeled and cut into thin rounds

SERVES 1

lime and mint spritzer

Cleansing on the palate, this citrus-infused refresher makes a great summer drink.

1 lemon

2 limes

½ teaspoon sugar (optional)

chilled tonic water or sparkling mineral water

crushed ice

slices of lemon and lime

10 fresh mint leaves

SERVES 2

Use a citrus press or hand-held juicer to squeeze the juice from the lemon and limes into a jug. Stir in the sugar, if using. Divide between 2 tall glasses and top up with tonic water.

Add crushed ice, slices of lemon and lime, and mint leaves before serving.

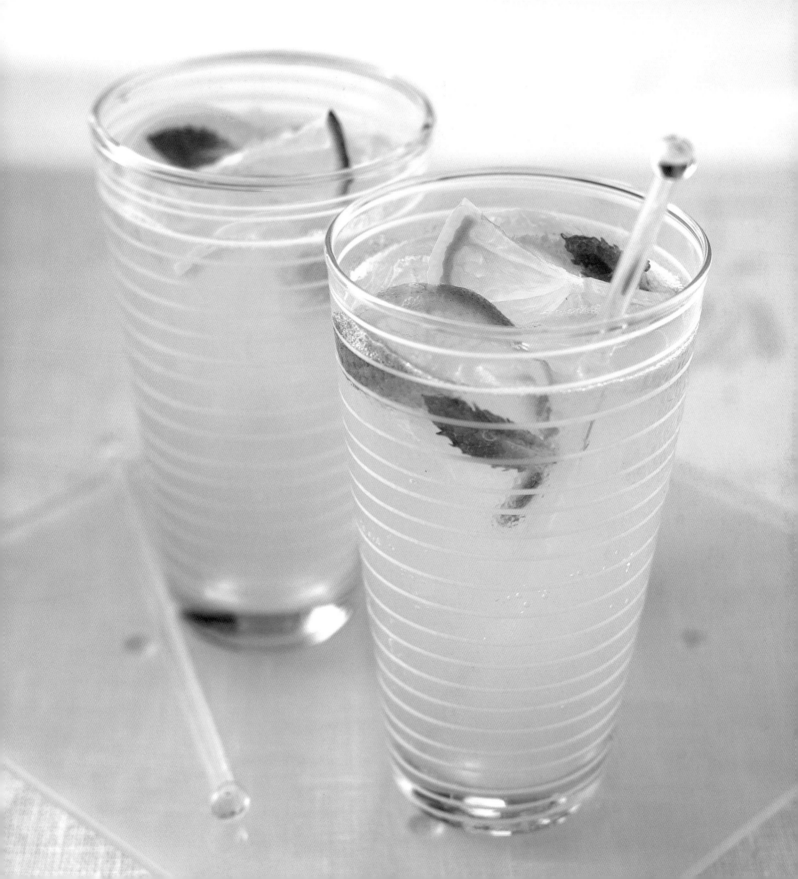

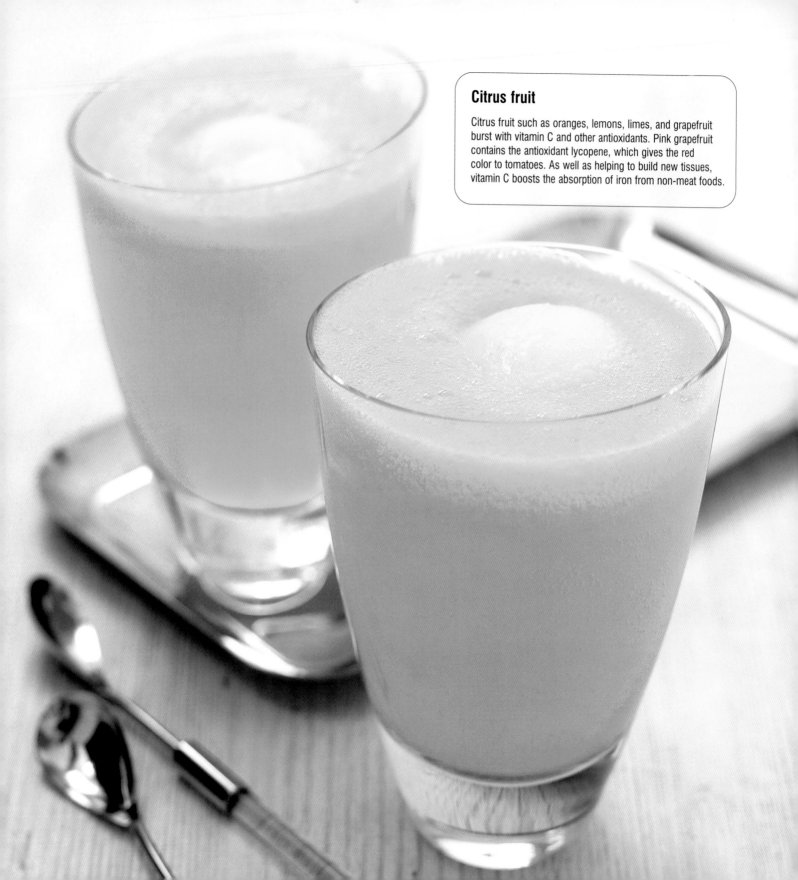

Citrus fruit

Citrus fruit such as oranges, lemons, limes, and grapefruit burst with vitamin C and other antioxidants. Pink grapefruit contains the antioxidant lycopene, which gives the red color to tomatoes. As well as helping to build new tissues, vitamin C boosts the absorption of iron from non-meat foods.

citrus fizz

This refreshing cooler is perfect if you are feeling overheated or need a quick pick-me-up. It is packed with vitamin C, one of the key nutrients that you need more of during pregnancy.

Use a citrus press or hand-held juicer to squeeze the juice from the oranges and grapefruit. Pour the juice through a strainer into 2 tall glasses and add a squeeze of lemon juice to each one.

Add a large scoop of lemon sorbet to each glass and top up with sparkling mineral water. Serve with a long-handled spoon.

5 oranges, halved horizontally

1 red or pink grapefruit, halved horizontally

a squeeze of fresh lemon juice

2 large scoops of lemon sorbet

chilled sparkling mineral water, to serve

SERVES 2

mango and lime lassi

Great with spicy food or as a satisfying snack, this soothing, cooling drink contains an abundance of beta-carotene (which the body converts to vitamin A), vitamin C, and other antioxidants.

1 mango

½ cup thick, plain low-fat yogurt

1–2 teaspoons sugar

1¼ cups low-fat milk

a squeeze of fresh lime juice, to taste

ice cubes, to serve

SERVES 2

Cut the mango in half either side of the central pit. Taking the 2 halves, cut the flesh into a criss-cross pattern down to the skin. Press each half inside out, then cut the mango cubes away from the skin.

Put the mango in a blender with ½ cup water. Add the yogurt, sugar, and milk, then blend until smooth and creamy.

Add a squeeze of lime juice, to taste. Serve in 2 tall glasses with plenty of ice.

Mango and papaya

Transport yourself to the tropics with these luscious and versatile fruits, packed with beta-carotene, vitamin C, and other beneficial antioxidants. Enjoy them on their own for breakfast, or in fruit, rice, or green salads or a salsa, or puréed in drinks.

tropical fruit and cardamom lassi

Aromatic cardamom is a traditional digestive aid, while yogurt and the form of fiber found in bananas may help the natural balance of the digestive system.

4 green cardamom pods

1 mango

2 bananas, thickly sliced

6 tablespoons canned reduced-fat coconut milk

⅔ cup thick, plain low-fat yogurt

⅔ cup low-fat milk

ice cubes, to serve

SERVES 2

Remove the seeds from the cardamom pods and grind them to a coarse powder in a pestle and mortar.

Cut the mango in half either side of the central pit. Taking the 2 halves, cut the flesh into a criss-cross pattern down to the skin. Press each half inside out, then cut the mango cubes away from the skin.

Put the cardamom in a blender with the mango, bananas, coconut milk, yogurt, and milk, then blend until smooth and frothy—you may need to do this in 2 batches. Put ice cubes into 2 tall glasses and top up with the lassi.

no-booze piña colada

It can be difficult to find tasty non-alcoholic drinks. The delicious blend of ingredients in this cocktail is delightfully indulgent, but also supplies protein, vitamins, and minerals.

1 papaya

1 small pineapple

1 banana, thickly sliced

¾ cup canned reduced-fat coconut milk

⅔ cup thick, natural low-fat bio yogurt

SERVES 2

Cut the papaya in half, then scoop out the seeds with a spoon. Peel the papaya and cut into chunks. Cut the pineapple lengthwise into quarters, then cut away the skin, remove the core, and cut into chunks.

Put the papaya, pineapple, and banana in a blender with the coconut milk and yogurt, then blend until smooth and creamy—you may have to do this in 2 batches.

Yogurt

Low-fat yogurt is great for protein, B vitamins, zinc, bone-building calcium, and phosphorus, and provides "friendly" bacteria that can help to maintain a healthy balance in your digestive system. It is safe to eat during pregnancy, and makes a low-fat alternative to cream, ice cream, or crème fraîche.

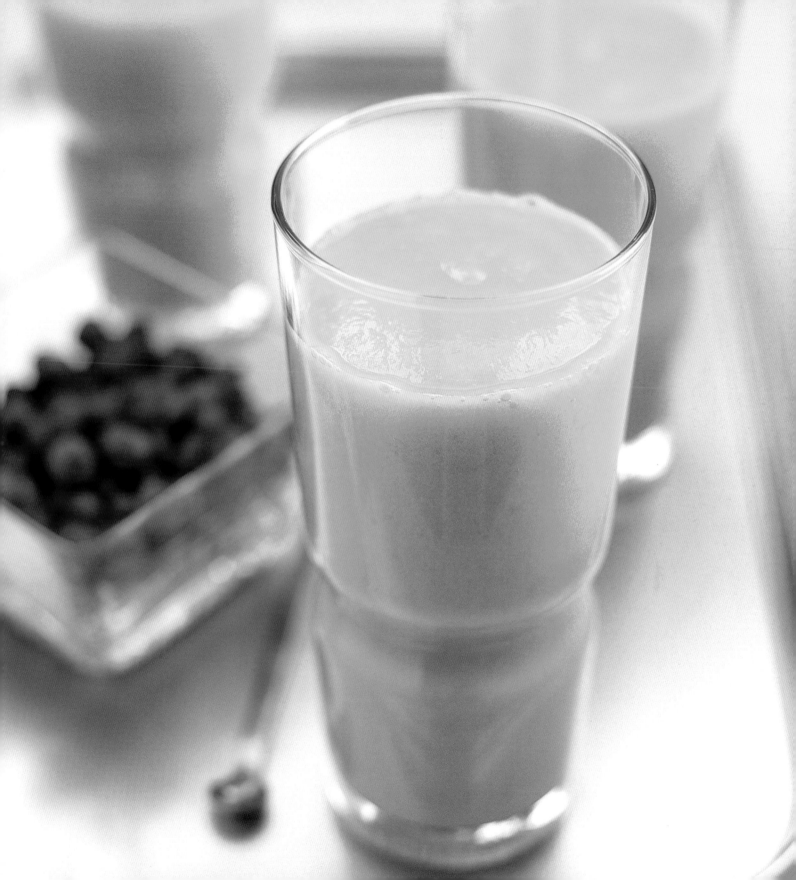

Index

Conversion chart

Weights and measures have been rounded up
or down slightly to make measuring easier.

Measuring butter:
A US stick of butter weighs 4 oz which is approximately
115 g or 8 tablespoons.

The recipes in this book require the following conversions:

American	Metric	Imperial
6 tbsp	85 g	3 oz
7 tbsp	100 g	3½ oz
1 stick	115 g	4 oz

Volume equivalents:

American	Metric	Imperial
1 teaspoon	5 ml	
1 tablespoon	15 ml	
¼ cup	60 ml	2 fl oz
⅓ cup	75 ml	2½ fl oz
½ cup	125 ml	4 fl oz
⅔ cup	150 ml	5 fl oz (¼ pint)
¾ cup	175 ml	6 fl oz
1 cup	250 ml	8 fl oz

Weight equivalents:

Imperial	Metric
1 oz	30 g
2 oz	55 g
3 oz	85 g
3½ oz	100 g
4 oz	115 g
6 oz	175 g
8 oz (½ lb)	225 g
9 oz	250 g
10 oz	280 g
12 oz	350 g
13 oz	375 g
14 oz	400 g
15 oz	425 g
16 oz (1 lb)	450 g

Measurements:

Inches	cm
¼ inch	5 mm
½ inch	1 cm
1 inch	2.5 cm
2 inches	5 cm
3 inches	7 cm
4 inches	10 cm
5 inches	12 cm
6 inches	15 cm
7 inches	18 cm
8 inches	20 cm
9 inches	23 cm
10 inches	25 cm
11 inches	28 cm
12 inches	30 cm

Oven temperatures:

120°C	(250°F)	Gas ½
140°C	(275°F)	Gas 1
150°C	(300°F)	Gas 2
170°C	(325°F)	Gas 3
180°C	(350°F)	Gas 4
190°C	(375°F)	Gas 5
200°C	(400°F)	Gas 6
220°C	(425°F)	Gas 7

Useful addresses

March of Dimes
1275 Mamaroneck Avenue
White Plains
NY 10605
Tel: (914) 997-4488
www.marchofdimes.com

**American Dietetic
Association**
120 Riverside Plaza
Suite 2000
Chicago, IL 69696-6995
Tel: 800/877-1600
eatright.org

Baby Center
163 Freelon Street
San Francisco, CA 94107
Tel: (866) 710-2229
www.babycenter.com/pregnancy

**La Leche League
International**
957 N. Plum Grove Road
Schaumburg, IL 60173
www.llli.org

Acknowledgments

A big thank you to Nicola Graimes and everyone at Ryland
Peters & Small—it's been a real pleasure. Also to Fiona
Ford at the Centre for Pregnancy Nutrition, University of
Sheffield, for her expertise. And to my wonderful husband
Steve for his endless love and support.

Lyndel Costain

My sincere thanks go to Alison Starling, Catherine Osborne,
Toni Kay, and the rest of the team at Ryland Peters &
Small—it has been a pleasure to work with you all. I would
also like to thank my co-author, Lyndel Costain, for her
invaluable advice, guidance, and for being a great partner.

Nicola Graimes